YOU CAN DO SOMETHING
ABOUT YOUR
ALLERGIES

Also by Nelson Lee Novick, M.D.

Saving Face:
A Dermatologist's Guide to Maintaining a Healthier
and Younger Looking Face

Skin Care for Teens

Super Skin:
A Leading Dermatologist's Guide to
the Latest Breakthroughs in Skin Care

Baby Skin:
A Leading Dermatologist's Guide to Infant and
Childhood Skin Care

YOU CAN DO SOMETHING ABOUT YOUR

ALLERGIES

A LEADING DOCTOR'S GUIDE TO ALLERGY PREVENTION AND TREATMENT

NELSON LEE NOVICK, M.D.

A LISA DREW BOOK

Macmillan Publishing Company

NEW YORK

Maxwell Macmillan Canada

TORONTO

Maxwell Macmillan International

NEW YORK   OXFORD   SINGAPORE   SYDNEY

Lisa Drew Books
Macmillan Publishing Company
866 Third Avenue
New York, NY 10022

Maxwell Macmillan Canada, Inc.
1200 Eglinton Avenue East
Suite 200
Don Mills, Ontario M3C 3N1

Macmillan Publishing Company is part of the Maxwell Communication Group of Companies.

Library of Congress Cataloging-in-Publication Data
Novick, Nelson Lee.
You can do something about your allergies/Nelson Novick.
    p. cm.
"A Lisa Drew book."
ISBN 0-02-590785-9
1. Allergy—Popular works.   I. Title
RC585.N68 1994
616.97—dc20   93–832957
                                                          CIP

Macmillan books are available at special discounts for bulk purchases for sales promotions, premiums, fund-raising, or educational use. For details, contact:
Special Sales Director
Macmillan Publishing Company
866 Third Avenue
New York, NY 10022

Designed by Michael Mendelsohn

10 9 8 7 6 5 4 3 2 1

Printed in the United States of America

To my wife, Meryl,
and my five sons, Yoni, Yoel,
Ariel, Donny, and Avi,
for their love and support,
and for just being there in my life.

SPECIAL THANKS
To my office manager, Barbara Jerabek,
for her invaluable suggestions and criticisms
in the preparation of this book, and
to Lisa Drew for her encouragement
in my writing career
and her confidence in me over the years.

CONTENTS

PREFACE

llergy remedies are big business. Each year, particularly in the spring and autumn, we are barraged in the print and electronic media with advertisements and commercials for decongestants, antihistamines, and poison ivy creams. The lay press and popular self-help books alike are replete with all kinds of non-medicinal recommendations for allergy prevention and treatment, including dietary changes, vitamin supplementation, the use of special ionizers, acupuncture, chiropractic, stress reduction methods, biofeedback therapies, and even moving to Arizona. For most allergy sufferers the choices can make their heads spin, and in an often frenzied pursuit of relief they annually spend billions of dollars. But what actually are allergies, and does anything really work for them?

Practically every minute of every day for as long as you live, your body is under assault by a hostile environment. The world in which you work and play is filled with dirt, grease, grime, pollutants, cosmetics, untold numbers of bacteria, viruses, and fungi, as well as all kinds of other nasty parasites and critters just waiting to get at you. In your defense the body has evolved a complex, interrelated network of cells, tissues, glands, and other organs, collectively known as the *immune system*. This marvelous system works to prevent entry of all types of harmful invaders and roots out and destroys any that have managed to gain entry. Without such a surveillance and defense system, it wouldn't be very long before all of us succumbed to all kinds of illnesses.

Sometimes, for reasons that are not yet understood, this same immune system that is meant to sustain us becomes overly reactive to certain, usually harmless, substances. It may begin, for example, to hyperreact to such relatively innocent things as pollens, dust, and dander as though they were vicious enemies intent on harming us. Or it may respond alarmingly to ordinary foods or medications intended to help us rather than simply ignoring them. Such an immune system malfunction is known as *hypersensitivity* or *allergy*, and inflammation of the skin and mucous membranes, generally resulting in redness, irritation, itching, swelling, and tenderness, is the unhappy result.

The particular kinds of allergy symptoms you suffer from naturally depend on the specific organs involved in the allergy attack. Symptoms can range from annoying to downright incapacitating or, at times, even life-threatening. Common allergy sites include the eyes, nose, throat, lungs, digestive tract, and skin.

Not surprisingly, allergies are nothing new to mankind. In fact, descriptions of allergy attacks extend back to the beginnings of recorded history. Ancient Egyptian documents and those of other early civilizations attest to a recognition of allergic disorders even in those days.

Today, it is estimated, there are over 40 million allergy sufferers in the United States alone, and allergies continue to be among the leading causes of both acute and chronic disease. In children they are responsible for more absences from school than any other medical condition, and in adults, for a substantial loss of productivity. Tragically, several hundred Americans die each year from severe allergic reactions.

It is for the weary, often exasperated allergy sufferer that *You Can Do Something About Your Allergies* has been written. Beginning with a brief description of the immune system and its relation to allergic reactions, the book covers a broad range of common allergic diseases. Attention is given to seasonal and perennial allergies, asthma, food and drug sensitivities, cosmetic and plant reactions, pollution and other environmentally related problems, and hypersensitivity responses to all kinds of stings and bites. Emphasis has been given to detailing proven ways to allergy-proof the home, to prevent allergy attacks outdoors, and to alleviate symptoms once underway. A special effort has been made to separate fact from fancy about many popular (and some little-known) allergy tests and treatments. First-aid measures are detailed for coping with anaphylaxis, or life-threatening, allergy attacks. A chapter is also devoted to the less well known problem of autoimmune diseases, those conditions in which the immune system attacks the body itself as though it were a foreign invader. The book centers not only on what your doctor can do for you but also, just as important, what you can do for yourself in the way of allergy prevention and home therapy.

Finally, for convenience, two appendices have been provided. The first appendix summarizes some of the tests used in determining allergic disorders, such as scratch tests, intradermal testing, RAST, and patch tests. The second appendix reviews the medications and treatments frequently prescribed for allergic disorders. In addition to listing the active ingredients and discussing the rationales for the suggested medications, specific brand name recommendations are made whenever available.

The products mentioned throughout the book are ones with which I have had considerable personal experience and have found to be consistently effective; however, I am not endorsing any product or products or any generic substance. In many instances the products mentioned are not the only ones available for dealing with the conditions discussed, and exclusion from the list of recommended items does imply that a particular product is not as effective. Where some products or therapies have been found worthless, I clearly say so. I do suggest, however, that you consult a physician if you have any questions about the value or efficacy of a specific drug or therapy.

Finally, given the nature of this book, the descriptions and explanations of medical therapies and techniques must be addressed to the general concerns of a wide audience. If you have particular questions or concerns about a medication or a form of therapy described in this book, you should of course consult your doctor. And should you require medical attention, the information contained in this volume will enable you to be a more knowledgeable, more confident participant in your own allergy health care.

You *Can* Do Something About Your Allergies.

CHAPTER ONE

WHAT'S IT ALL ABOUT?
THE BASICS OF ALLERGIES

D o you wake up each morning with your nose so stuffed you can hardly breathe? Do you break out in hives every time you eat nuts? Is your skin so sensitive that no matter what cream or soap you use, you develop a rash? If these questions ring a familiar bell, you're not alone. Hardly a day goes by in my private practice that at least one patient doesn't express concern that he or she may be suffering from an allergy. For example, patients often want to know if their headaches, skin rashes, or sinus problems represent an allergy to something they've come in contact with or eaten. Frequently they bring with them a shopping list of what they think may be the cause of their troubles—specific germs, foods, cosmetics, medications. Much of the time these concerns are based on misinformation obtained from friends or the media.

Concerns about allergies to *Candida,* the common intestinal yeast organism best known for causing one form of vaginitis in women, are a good example of this. Because of the bad publicity the organism has received lately, patients with no evidence of *Candida* infection at all will ask whether their complaints of chronic fatigue, psoriasis, or migraines can be due to overcolonization by the organism. In a similar vein, other patients will relate some of all of their symptoms to environmental pollution or food contaminants.

Whatever the realities regarding the role of *Candida* or environmental pollution in triggering allergic disorders, one thing is sure: Allergies are of no small medical and consumer concern. More people see physicians for the relief of allergy symptoms than for any other single illness. It has been estimated that approximately one-fifth of the population of the Western world suffers with some form of allergy. It is so common, in fact, that almost everyone personally knows someone who suffers from them. In the United States alone, more than $100 million is spent each year for allergy injections. And to the delight of the pharmaceutical industry, allergy sufferers spend nearly $500 million annually on an overwhelming array of over-the-counter remedies in search of relief.

To obtain the kind of care you need and to avoid being misled by advertising claims or bogus therapies, you need to know more about what allergies are, what triggers them, and what you can do about them.

WHAT IS AN ALLERGY?

Simply put, an allergy is an abnormal reaction to one or more substances or environmental conditions that are harmless to most other people. For this reason doctors often refer to allergy attacks as *hypersensitivity* reactions (that is, an oversensitivity to something). The fact that allergies often run in families suggests that the predisposition to develop them is inherited.

As a rule, allergy attacks do not begin by themselves; they are triggered by exposure to *antigens* or *allergens*. These typically are water-soluble proteins capable of penetrating the mucous membranes or skin barrier. Common allergens include tree pollens, weeds, and grasses, house dust, molds, animal dander, insect parts or venom, certain foods and drugs, and paint, perfume, and solvent fumes. (These and other types of allergies, along with the contributory role of environmental conditions—heat, cold, humidity, sunlight, and pollution—will be discussed later.)

Becoming Allergic to Something

Contrary to a popular misconception, an allergy attack is typically *not* provoked by the first exposure to a particular allergen. Instead, a person actually becomes *sensitized* (that is, becomes allergic) to a substance following repeated exposures to it over a period of weeks, months, or even years. In fact, allergy symptoms may not develop until after the tenth, hundredth, or even thousandth exposure. Doctors refer to this interval as the period of sensitization. Once an individual has become sensitized, however, allergy symptoms, in most cases, will develop each time the susceptible person is exposed to the offending allergen. In general, once a person is allergic to something, it takes only a minute or trace amount of the allergen to trigger symptoms.

ALLERGY ATTACKS AND THE IMMUNE SYSTEM

To better understand what goes on during a typical allergy attack, you first need to know a few basic facts about your immune system, which is responsible for allergies. In healthy people the immune system is the body's natural defense network against invasion by parasites, fungi, bacteria, and viruses. In addition, it functions to root out and destroy other unwanted "parasites," such as malignancies, in their very early stages, before they have a chance to spread. In fact, without a properly functioning immune system, we would all surely die from a host of infections and cancers. It is precisely for this reason that victims of AIDS, who suffer from severely compromised immune function, succumb to various types of infections and malignant tumors that do not ordinarily affect healthy (that is, immunologically normal) individuals.

Although a listing of only the most common allergens in our environment would fill many books, there are just three main routes for them to gain access to the body. They may be inhaled, swallowed, or absorbed through the skin and mucous membranes. This information is important since it is the route the allergens take that determines the symptoms a person suffers. Pollens, house dust, and chemical fumes, for example, are inhaled and therefore trigger the stuffy head, runny nose, and sneezing of hay fever and other respiratory allergies. Foods and drugs taken by mouth can give rise to local gastrointestinal symptoms, and once absorbed through the intestines into the bloodstream, they are capable of causing widespread allergic reactions such as hives. Following direct contact with the skin, certain plants, such as the all-too-familiar poison ivy, typically precipitate an intensely itchy, blistering, and oozing eruption. Finally, by injecting toxins or other substances into the skin (which eventually reach the bloodstream), a multitude of stinging or biting insects may provoke local hivelike reactions or severe systemic allergic symptoms, such as respiratory difficulty, hypertension, and shock.

Regardless of where allergies take place in the body or what the specific symptoms are, allergic reactions result from the reaction to the substance by one or more of the three major components of the immune system: (1) cells known as *lymphocytes, plasma cells*, and *mast cells*, (2) particular types of proteins called *antibodies*, and (3) a variety of chemical substances known as *mediators*.

Specialized Cells and Chemical Mediators

Since immunity and allergy are but two faces of the immune system, you should not be surprised to learn that both kinds of reactions involve many of the same elements. Lymphocytes, for example, are among the specialized white blood cells called into action in both allergic and ordinary immune reactions. One type, the *T lymphocyte*, works by surrounding foreign invaders or allergens and secreting chemical mediators capable of both destroying the invader and of recruiting additional white blood cells to the affected area to join the battle.

In response to allergens or other foreign materials, a second type of lymphocyte, the *B lymphocyte*, is also often enlisted. Once stimulated, B lymphocytes undergo internal changes to become a new kind of cell, known as a plasma cell, that possesses the ability to manufacture and secrete antibodies into the blood. Antibodies are special types of proteins that work by binding tightly to invading germs or allergens, inactivating them and speeding their removal from the body.

Three other cells, *eosinophils*, *basophils*, and *mast cells*, also figure prominently in immune reactions and allergy. Eosinophils are specialized white blood cells that, under ordinary circumstances, are important for battling large-sized foreign invaders, particularly parasitic worms. However, for reasons that remain unclear, they are also produced in large numbers in certain allergic disorders, especially hay fever. In fact, they are so often seen under the microscope in the nasal and bronchial mucus secretions of hay fever and asthma sufferers that they are commonly referred to by doctors as "allergy cells."

Basophils are another form of white blood cell. Found both in the bloodstream and near the surface of the mucous membranes lining the eyes and nose, these cells contain many kinds of chemical mediators. Some mediators are stored within the cell, and others are produced in response to allergenic stimulation. They are responsible for many tissue changes; for example, they are capable of dilating small blood vessels, stimulating the tiny nerve endings in the mucous membranes, promoting mucus production, and stimulating other tissues to become involved in the overall inflammatory process.

Mast cells are another extremely important type of allergy cell. Ordinarily located deep in the linings of the nose and eyes, these cells typically accumulate in close proximity to blood vessels and mucus-producing cells. Like basophils, mast cells are producers and storers of a wide variety of very potent chemical mediators. They also share with basophils a special affinity for binding IgE molecules (discussed below) to their outer surfaces, a step crucial in the evolution of many types of allergy attacks.

Of the dozen or so mediators so far discovered, *histamine* is probably best known. Among its many effects, it is responsible for dilating small blood vessels and provoking the inflammation and swelling of tissues. Histamine is believed to provoke such diverse symptoms as the stuffiness, the mucous discharge, and the constricted passageways characteristic of hay fever and asthma attacks and the itchiness of eczemas. For this reason antihistamines—drugs that, as the term implies, block the effects of histamine—make up an important part of our arsenal of anti-allergy therapies.

Antibodies

Often referred to as *gamma globulins* or *immunoglobulins*, antibodies are divided into five main classes. By far the most common variety is *immunoglobulin G*, otherwise known as IgG. IgG antibodies in the bloodstream are largely responsible for the protection produced by immunizations, such as those against measles and rubella.

Immunoglobulin A (IgA), which is found in stomach and nasal secretions and in breast milk, is the second class of immunoglobulins. IgA serves as the first line of defense against attack to the mucus membranes of the respiratory and digestive tracts.

The third class of immunoglobulins, immuniglobulin E, IgE, is a major weapon in your body's natural defense against assault by large organisms, such as parasitic worms. To allergy sufferers, however, this antibody is better known for its critical role in sensitizing people to specific allergens and for inducing allergy attacks (discussed below). For these reasons IgE has earned the dubious reputation of being the primary allergy antibody.

Immediate and Delayed Hypersensitivity Reactions

Immunologists, physicians, and researchers who deal with the immune system and diseases of immunity generally divide allergic reactions into two major categories: immediate and delayed. Immediate reactions, also called Type I reactions, occur soon after exposure to an offending allergen, usually within one to four hours.

Immediate hypersensitivity generally involves IgE antibodies. Hay fever is a common example of this form of reaction.

Delayed responses, on the other hand, may occur as much as two to five days after exposure, sometimes even longer. Rather than antibodies, other kinds of cells, particularly T-lymphocytes, are believed to be the prime movers in this type of allergy reaction. Delayed responses are generally referred to as Type IV reactions. The poison ivy rash is a well-known example.

INITIAL SENSITIZATION AND SUBSEQUENT REEXPOSURES

With this background in mind, you are now able to understand what goes on when you become initially sensitized (that is, allergic) to a specific allergen and what is involved in triggering subsequent allergy attacks at each individual encounter with your allergenic nemesis. To appreciate sensitization—the process of developing an allergy—let's follow ordinary ragweed pollen grains, the bane of hay fever sufferers, after they enter the respiratory tract.

Once inside, the tiny grains quickly make contact with plasma cells located in the tissues and tiny blood vessels. In response, these cells immediately begin producing IgE antibodies capable of targeting the ragweed pollens. Once produced, the IgE molecules in turn bind to the thousands of surrounding mast cells and basophils to which they have a natural affinity. Somewhere between one hundred to three hundred thousand ragweed-specific IgE molecules may coat each mast cell or basophil. Once this binding process is complete, whether it occurs after the first exposure or the thousandth, the individual is thereafter sensitized to ragweed—or, if you prefer, allergic to it.

Now let's examine what happens when a previously sensitized individual (that is, one who is already allergic) is exposed once more to the substance to which he has become allergic. We'll use ragweed as an example again. Once they enter the respiratory system of a hay fever sufferer, the pollens immediately bind to the many IgE molecules on the surfaces of the mast cells and basophils, activating them and triggering the release of many types of chemical mediators, including histamine. When this occurs, symptoms begin.

But that's not the end of the story. Several hours later, in what is called the *late-phase* reaction, eosinophils and additional basophils become attracted to the allergy site, and these latecomers contribute not only to the severity of the symptoms but to the persistence of the attack. The result of all these processes in our example is the sneezing, runny nose, congestion, and watery eyes of a typical immediate hypersensitivity hay fever attack.

Although constituting by far the most common type of antibody-related allergic reactions, IgE (Type I) allergies are not the only kinds of antibodies responsible for allergy attacks. IgM and IgG antibodies, the body's two major infection-fighting antibodies, are involved in what are called Type II allergy reactions, which involve a slight variation in the steps just described. In these instances, allergens bind first to a specific target tissue (such as red blood corpuscles or platelets), and it is the allergen-cell complex that then attracts the antibodies and results in cellular destruction. Overall, these varieties of allergic reaction, also called *cytotoxic* reactions because they lead to damage and destruction of cells, are quite rare. When they do occur, they are often linked to the use of sulfa drugs and quinidine.

Type III reactions are the third kind of antibody-mediated allergic responses. Also known as *serum sickness disease*, these reactions, which also involve IgM and IgG antibodies, differ from the Type II responses in that the antibodies and the allergens bind directly with each other in the bloodstream to form floating allergen-antibody complexes. Eventually these relatively large circulating clumps become trapped in the networks of tiny blood vessels found in the kidneys, lungs, joints, and skin, where they are capable of triggering considerable inflammation and tissue damage.

Finally, in the case of delayed allergic reactions (Type IV), the process of sensitization itself is somewhat different from that described earlier. In Type IV reactions, antibodies are not involved. Rather, direct contact with an allergen, such as poison ivy, induces the development of the allergy by bringing about a permanent alteration in the cell surfaces of T lymphocytes. Once this alteration has taken place, each subsequent reexposure to the offending allergen provokes the sensitized T cells to release the chemical mediators responsible for the itchy, blistering skin rash that results.

HOW DO ALLERGIES DIFFER FROM NORMAL IMMUNE RESPONSES?

Technically, an allergy is an *abnormal* immune response. It differs from normal immune reactions in two main ways. First, it is triggered by basically harmless substances, such as pollens, rather than by germs or other threatening organisms or cancers. Second, it tends to be prolonged and out of proportion to what is actually needed to dispose of the offending substance. By contrast, normal immune responses generally match the problem at hand and last no longer than are needed to do the job.

IT'S NOT IN YOUR HEAD

One point should be clear from the foregoing: Allergies are true physical disorders arising from complex chemical and physical interactions between allergens, specialized cells, antibodies, and chemical mediators. And while allergies are often responsible for a good deal of emotional suffering, they are not, contrary to a popular misconception, emotional diseases. No matter what you have heard, they are not "just in your head."

All the same, heightened nervous tension may play a role in certain allergies. The anxiety, fear, and emotional stress that allergies commonly engender in sufferers, for example, may contribute to the triggering of attacks or the aggravating of existing allergy symptoms, leading to a vicious cycle of suffering. For the many allergy victims who are known to have more than one allergy, the overall picture can be even worse.

Two Common Reactions That Are Often Confused with Allergies

True allergies must be distinguished from two other common medical problems with which they are often confused: *side effects* and *intolerance*. A side effect is a predictable reaction to a certain medication or food. Antihistamines serve as a good example. The grogginess they cause when taken is an expected side effect and is not an allergic reaction. In the same way, the flatulence experienced by many people after consuming beans is a side effect, not an allergic reaction.

An intolerance, on the other hand, is an *exaggeration* of an expected reaction to a particular food or medication. Continuing with the examples above, if you slept for sixteen hours after taking one antihistamine tablet or if you experienced excessive gas, cramping, or diarrhea after consuming a normal-sized portion of beans, it would be correct to say that you are demonstrating an intolerance to these substances, not an allergy.

The difference between side effects, intolerances, and true allergies is more than academic. Let's say you are aware that you cannot tolerate penicillin, that it gives you stomach cramps. Regardless of that reaction, if you needed penicillin to cure you of some serious infection, you could still safely take it when no satisfactory substitute is available (and suffer the expected cramps). On the other hand, if you developed allergic, life-threatening respiratory problems from taking penicillin, you would not be able to take it. Clearly, then, recognizing the difference between an allergy and a side effect or intolerance can be extremely important and even life-saving.

Do You Have Allergies?

Now that we have some ideas about allergies, how do you know whether allergies are your problems? If you are unsure, you might ask yourself the following questions, which can serve as a guide. A "yes" answer to any of them *may* indicate an allergic basis for your complaints.

An Allergy Quiz
1. Do you suffer from hives?
2. Do you get frequent itchy skin rashes?
3. Do you get localized areas of skin swellings or bumpiness?
4. Do you suffer with migraine or other headaches?
5. Do you complain of chronic fatigue that is not alleviated by sleep?
6. Do you complain of red, itchy, or watery eyes?
7. Do you have dark rings or swelling around your eyes?
8. Do you have trouble with your contact lenses?
9. Are your ears frequently stuffed or popping?
10. Do you complain of catching frequent "colds"?
11. Do you suffer with sinus congestion?
12. Do you have a constant postnasal drip?
13. Is your nose always stuffed or running?
14. Do you have frequent nosebleeds?
15. Do you snore heavily at night or have other nightly breathing problems?
16. Do you find your sense of taste or smell dulled?
17. Do you wheeze?
18. Are you troubled by a constant cough?
19. Are you annoyed by a tickle in your throat?
20. Do you suffer with bloating, frequent abdominal cramping, nausea, or diarrhea?

A few words to the wise are in order: Since each of the above complaints may also be caused by a variety of nonallergic disorders, it would be prudent to seek the advice of a qualified physician to determine the precise cause(s) of your problem.

DON'T DELAY SEEKING HELP!

There are no advantages to delaying the search for medical help. To the contrary, early diagnosis and treatment of allergies are now thought to be important not only for alleviating symptoms but for preventing potential complications. Nor should you be fooled into thinking your allergy is getting better by itself. Although you may have periods when the symptoms wax and wane, allergies as a rule are not "outgrown." In fact, the reverse is true: In the vast majority of instances, allergies tend to worsen with time.

In addition, you should not discount the possibility that you have an allergy just because you never had one before. Symptoms can begin at any age, not just in the early years as some people mistakenly believe.

Although medical science has not yet reached the stage where it is possible to alter the genes responsible for the development of allergies, an attack can be made on the genetic basis for most allergic conditions. You will discover as you read further that there are many effective ways to control and treat allergic manifestations. Happily, you need not suffer from allergies, and therefore you really can and should do something about them.

CHAPTER TWO

THE AIR CAN BE TEEMING WITH TROUBLE: SEASONAL ALLERGIC RHINITIS

Ah, it's springtime again, when young people's fancies turn to romance and to fun outdoors. Right? Wrong! Not for the more than one in every twenty people who suffer from "rose fever," or grass or tree pollen allergies. The suffering is no less intense for the countless others who are plagued by summer and autumn "hay fever" allergies. Correctly known as seasonal allergic rhinitis, these allergies are responsible for millions of days of absenteeism from work and school and millions of days of bed rest and restricted activity by otherwise healthy people every year. (Perennial allergic rhinitis—allergic rhinitis that persists year-round—is the subject of the next chapter.)

The term hay fever, which is hundreds of years old, originated when certain individuals became very ill every year during the English hay-pitching season. The term is misleading, however. For one thing, the condition has more to do with the grasses that pollinate during hay-pitching season than to the hay itself. For another, there is no fever associated with the condition. To avoid these inaccuracies, physicians prefer the term *allergic rhinitis,* or allergy-induced nasal inflammation, for all seasonal allergies. Because the term covers more of the sufferer's symptoms, physicians sometimes use the tongue-twister *allergic rhinoconjunctivitis,* which simply means allergically-induced nasal and eye irritations.

TYPICAL SIGNS AND SYMPTOMS

Although a first episode of allergic rhinitis may take place at any age (even in one's eighties), it most commonly occurs in the teen years, particularly between the ages of twelve and fifteen. The symptoms may be maddening at times and often include severe nasal congestion and stuffiness, and fits of sneezing. Ten or more sneezes at a time are not uncommon. Victims may also have a profuse watery mucus discharge and an annoying postnasal drip. To make matters worse, intense itching in and around the nose, on the roof of the mouth, and deep within the ears is also common. Younger children who have these itchy-nosed allergies exhibit the characteristic "fingers pointing upward and palm flat against the nose" position of the hand, commonly called the "allergic salute" by pediatricians.

Other symptoms include a sore, scratchy, or itchy throat; red, itchy, watery eyes; and inflammation of the conjunctiva, the membrane that protects the eye. Congestion of the *eustachian tubes*, small canal-like structures that connect the middle ear with the area in back of the nose and throat, can result in an annoying feeling of ear pressure—the kind you experience when changing altitudes in a plane—and diminished hearing. It may even give rise to an outright earache. Finally, victims may suffer with headaches and complain of fatigue and irritability. In general, on any given day the severity of the symptoms of seasonal allergic rhinitis depends on the amount of pollen in the air and, of course, on the degree of sensitivity of the individual. (The relationship between seasonal allergies and the development of asthma, a more serious respiratory condition, is discussed in Chapter 5.)

Many of the common signs and symptoms are easily explainable. Nasal swelling, congestion, runny nose, and loss of smell and taste are believed to be the result of histamine (as well as other mediators) via its effects on blood vessels and tissues. As in the case of the common cold, the diminished sense of taste and smell are explained by the fact that excessive secretions interfere with contact between the tiny molecules of food or fragrances and the tips of the nerves responsible for taste and smell perception.

Red, itchy, swollen, and watery eyes are likewise believed to be linked to the release of histamine by mast cells within the delicate membranes of the conjunctivae. Conscious or unconscious rubbing in response to the itching, which so often accompanies the symptoms, only worsens the redness and irritation. Not surprisingly, contact lens wearers have even a harder time because pollen particles trapped between the contact lens and the eye typically trigger numerous tiny allergic reactions. Not uncommonly, lens wearers have "bloodshot" eyes and complain of burning, grittiness, dryness, and significantly reduced lens comfort and wearing time.

The earaches and stuffed ears, as well as the crackling and popping sounds that commonly accompany allergic rhinitis, are also easily explained. Under ordinary circumstances, the eustachian tubes adjust to any changes in outside air pressure by opening and closing automatically. This occurs, for example, whenever you dive into water or ascend or descend in an elevator or airplane. When they are swollen from allergy, however, the eustachian tubes malfunction, giving rise to sensations of crackling and popping or painful pressure in the ears. If the problem persists, inflammatory fluid within the surrounding blood vessels may leak into the canals; if it accumulates sufficiently, it can lead to hearing difficulties and even secondary bacterial invasion.

VASOMOTOR RHINITIS

The common disorder known as vasomotor rhinitis must be distinguished from true allergic rhinitis. This condition shares many of the same symptoms with its allergic counterpart, including stuffy nasal passages, runny nose, and sneezing, but the underlying cause is believed to be, as the name suggests, a vasomotor problem— that is, an abnormality of nerve control over blood vessel dilation and constriction. Not uncommonly, it is triggered by physical factors, such as sharp changes in temperature or humidity, as well as by smoke, room odors, and pollution. For some reason even sunshine may precipitate bouts of reflex sneezing in some victims with this condition. Increased nervous tension can likewise play an aggravating role.

Unfortunately, vasomotor rhinitis is chronic and may persist year-round. Treatment is difficult, although in many instances relief may be obtained with the same remedies used to treat its allergic counterpart (as discussed below). Unfortunately, some individuals may have both problems, making matters that much worse.

WHAT IS "SINUS"?

People often refer to sinus, or sinus trouble, to denote chronic headache problems or pain and pressure behind the eyes or cheeks. Others use these terms to describe the nasal stuffiness of hay fever. *Sinusitis* is the correct medical term for all forms of inflammation involving any of the sinuses.

Everyone has four pairs of sinuses: The frontal sinuses are located above the eyes; the ethmoid sinuses are on the sides of the nose; the sphenoid sinuses are behind the ethmoids; and the maxillary sinuses are behind the cheekbones. All are mucous membrane–lined, air-filled cavities within the skull that lead into the nasal passages. Although their precise function is not known, they are believed to play a role in aerodynamically lightening the skull and in the reception of smells and sounds.

Experts estimate that nearly 70 percent of all chronic sinusitis cases are caused by allergies. Compounding the problem, many of these cases become secondarily infected by bacteria. Contrary to conventional wisdom, sinusitis is not just an adult problem. Children, too, may suffer from "sinus" conditions and their complications.

The headaches characteristic of sinus allergies are believed to be due to a blockage of the openings of the sinuses into the nose, caused by swollen nasal tissue, and the subsequent buildup of pressure in the sinuses. The pain is severest directly over the sinuses, and depending on which of the sinuses is most affected, it may be experienced in the forehead or directly behind or under the eyes. Due to the overnight accumulation of secretions within the sinus cavities and to the diminished ability to clear them, sinus headaches are typically worse when rising in the morning.

To complicate the picture, conditions within chronically allergic sinuses are ripe for bacterial invasion and pus formation. A change from clear to yellowish or greenish nasal secretions suggests bacterial infection. When this happens, sinus symptoms worsen. Postnasal dripping at the back of the throat may occur, additionally giving rise to throat irritation and coughing. More severe cases of sinusitis may be accompanied by fever, muscular aches, and even swelling and tenderness of the skin above the affected areas.

POLLENS AND MOLD SPORES

Pollens, the main troublemakers for most cases of seasonal allergic rhinitis, are actually microscopic, fertilizing, male cells in the reproductive cycle of many kinds of flowering plants and trees. Because of their minute size and extreme dryness, pollen grains are easily blown about by the wind and may be carried hundreds of miles by air currents. A single ragweed plant may discharge into the air as many as eight billion grains of pollen, and in a typical season more than a quarter of a million tons may blow about the countryside—to the dismay of allergy sufferers. This is why local small-scale destruction of ragweed plants usually has little effect overall in lessening the problem.

Mold, another very common respiratory allergen, is the microscopic form of a nonflowering parasitic plant life known as fungi. Like other forms of fungi, mold lacks roots, stems, leaves, and chlorophyll. As a result, it must obtain its nourishment from other plant and animal materials. Well-known for its ability to spoil foods, mold grows on corn, wheat, and oats; it is therefore a particular problem in the grain-producing regions of the Midwest. Molds propagate by producing spores, which, like pollens, are dispersed in huge numbers by the wind.

For the benefit of its local populace, many regional hospitals provide "pollen count" updates to the local radio and television stations.

A pollen count is a measurement of the number of pollen grains in each cubic yard of air collected in a twenty-four-hour period. Specially coated glass rods are used to capture the pollen grains, and special stains are used to identify them. Typical pollen counts during an average season may range from two hundred to five hundred, with readings of more than one hundred causing discomfort for the majority of allergy sufferers.

It is important to keep in mind that the pollen count heard on the morning news reflects the previous day's count and is not necessarily a prediction of what the new day will bring. Also, mold counts are sometimes obtained with the use of special gathering devices, but they are less commonly reported.

AN ALLERGY FOR ALL SEASONS

Although the infamous ragweed is responsible for the majority of cases, seasonal allergic rhinitis can also be caused by a wide variety of tree, grass, and weed pollens as well as by mold spores. Naturally, symptoms will be at their worst during the time of year that the particular plant to which you are allergic is pollinating.

Pollination occurs at different times in different parts of the country, but the following can serve as a general guideline for seasonal allergies. Springtime allergic rhinitis (February to May) may be caused by hypersensitivity to the pollens from ash, birch, cypress, elm, maple, oak, poplar, sycamore, and walnut trees. Midsummer allergies (April to mid-June) usually result from pollinating grasses, such as orchard grass, redtop, rye, timothy, sweet vernal grass, fescue, Johnson grass, and various bluegrasses, which are the most problematic allergen in the West. Finally, end-of-summer and early autumn allergies (mid-August to October) are mostly due to ragweed pollens and to the pollens of several closely related weeds: cosmos, golden glows, goldenrods, and zinnias.

Like hay fever, rose fever is another misnomer. In general, brightly colored and fragrant flowers such as roses do not rely on the wind to disperse their pollens. Instead, the generally sticky pollens they produce attach to birds, bees, and insects, which is how they are transferred from plant to plant. For that reason, bright and fragrant flowering plants are seldom the cause of seasonal allergic rhinitis.

Molds abound in most places in the world except for deserts. They are particularly common at the shores of seas and lakes. Outdoors, they may be found on decaying vegetation and wood, fresh-cut grass, piles of leaves, and compost heaps. They may also be found on a variety of vegetables, including corn, tomatoes, and sweet potatoes. The bulk of outdoor mold allergies are linked to two main spore producers: *Alternaria* and *Cladosporium (Hormodendrum)*. Depending on where you live, the height of the mold season may be anywhere from April to November.

Interestingly, the allergy to Christmas trees that many people suffer from may be caused by both molds and pollens. Both kinds of allergens are attached to the trees and remain there after the trees have been cut and stored. Indoor heat then releases the offending allergens, which accounts for the several-week-long December hay fever "season" experienced in many homes.

The weather may also play an important role in allergic rhinitis. In general, most people with seasonal allergic rhinitis caused by pollens fare better on cool, windless, muggy or rainy days because cool weather reduces pollination, and dampness makes pollen less aerodynamically efficient. By contrast, since warmth encourages pollination, hot, sunny, and especially windy days, with their ability to spew clouds of pollens or spores into the air, can be a curse for seasonal allergy sufferers.

The ability of molds to be dispersed by air currents in response to changes in temperature, humidity, and wind conditions is fairly similar to that seen with pollens. Consequently, mold suffers also do better on cool or rainy days. Unfortunately, molds may survive outdoors far longer than pollens, even during freezing weather. Troublesome spores may abound in stored hay, grain, and straw, causing year-round distress to mold-allergic farmers and other grain workers. For this reason we usually do not refer to a "mold season" the way we do to a "ragweed season."

Finally, there is one difficult-to-control environmental condition in which no one fares well, particularly allergy sufferers: air pollution. The combination of elevated levels of air pollution and high levels of molds and pollens spells misery for allergy sufferers.

DIAGNOSING AND TREATING SEASONAL ALLERGIC RHINITIS

The following briefly summarizes some of the more common methods of diagnosing and treating seasonal allergic rhinitis. Additional information can be found in Appendices A and B.

Diagnosis

Diagnosing the specific cause(s) of seasonal allergic rhinitis starts with a detailed history and physical examination by your doctor. Because so many allergy symptoms and signs can also be caused by nonallergic disorders such as infections, a deviated nasal septum, and nasal polyps, it is important to be sure that you are indeed suffering from an allergy rather than from some other condition.

The viral cold—or upper respiratory infection, as doctors often call it—is a common condition that must be differentiated from all forms of allergic rhinitis, including the seasonal variety. True colds produce many of the same symptoms as allergic rhinitis, but when these symptoms persist for several weeks and no other family members are affected, you are more likely to be suffering from an allergy. If your nasal problems are accompanied by a severe sore throat, muscle aches, and fever, however, you probably have an upper respiratory infection or the flu. (And, not surprisingly, poorly controlled allergic rhinitis appears to predispose some people to more frequent colds.)

Although the symptoms may be similar, the appearance of the mucous membranes of allergy sufferers differs from that of people with colds. The nasal mucosa, the lining of the nose, is typically pale and grayish in allergic disorders and the secretions are clear. By contrast, the mucosa tends to be an angry red and the secretions yellowish or greenish with true colds. The finding of so-called allergy cells, or eosinophils, in a sample of the nasal secretions is another helpful way to distinguish between the two conditions.

To confirm a suspected pollen or mold spore allergy and to pinpoint its specific cause(s), your doctor may order a variety of skin and blood tests. *Scratch tests*, which are used infrequently these days because of their lower rate of accuracy, consist of applying small dilutions of suspected allergens to tiny scratches made in the skin, usually of the forearm. The development of itching, redness, and hivelike swelling at a test site within fifteen to thirty minutes suggests an allergy to the test substance. *Intradermal tests*, which are used more frequently because of their greater accuracy, are similar to scratch tests except that the dilution of allergen is *injected* directly into the skin. Once again, redness, itching, and swelling indicate an allergy to a test material. After a particular allergen (or perhaps several) has been determined to be the culprit, skin tests may also be used to establish the best starting dose for desensitization (immunotherapy) therapy (which will be discussed below). Finally, a special blood test, known as the RAST, which looks for elevated levels of IgE in response to various allergens, may also be ordered.

Therapy

Therapy for seasonal allergic rhinitis may take several forms. The mainstays are the *antihistamines*. These medications, as their name suggests, block the effects of histamine on its target tissues, thereby reducing symptoms. More than six classes of antihistamines are available, and many—such as chlorpheniramine (**Chlor-Trimeton**) and diphenhydramine (**Benadryl**)—can be purchased over the counter (OTC), that is, without a doctor's prescription. Most have been around for many years and have a proven record of safety. Nevertheless, the older antihistamines often cause dryness and drowsiness, and many people cannot tolerate them for that reason. Other important side effects include urinary retention in men with enlarged prostates and aggravation of glaucoma. Two relatively newer antihistamines, astemizole (**Hismanal**) taken once daily, and terfenadine (**Seldane**) taken twice daily—both available by prescription only—have proven quite effective in controlling allergy symptoms without causing grogginess. And, finally, loratadine (**Claritin**), the newest prescription nonsedating antihistamine, combines the convenience of once daily dosing with rapid onset of action. Quite significantly, unlike the other two agents, it has not been reported to cause heart rhythm abnormalities when taken with either oral erythromycin or ketoconazole.

Decongestants, many of which are available without prescription, are another class of very useful products. These agents work to reduce congestion by constricting the tiny blood vessels in the affected areas, thereby reducing leakage of inflammatory fluid and minimizing swelling and itching. For this reason they are also known as *vasoconstrictors* (*vaso* means blood vessels). Decongestants have the added advantage of not causing grogginess.

Two of the more common decongestants include phenylpropanolamine, the active "upper" ingredient in many over-the-counter diet pills, and pseudoephedrine (**Sudafed**). Side effects may include nervousness, dizziness, headaches, and high blood pressure. Individuals with a history of hypertension, seizures, or stroke should consult with their physician before taking any of these medications.

Combination antihistamine and decongestant products abound on the shelves of our pharmacies and supermarkets. Some of the more well known brands are **Ornade, Allerest**, and **ARM**, which contain both chlorpheniramine and phenyl-propanolamine. Many people prefer such combinations not only for their two-pronged attack on symptoms but also because the stimulant effects of the decongestants serve to offset somewhat the drowsiness induced by the antihistamines. Nevertheless, doctors often recommend that their patients take separate antihistamine and decongestant tablets so that they may better regulate the exact amounts of each to control their effects. For those whose jobs or life-styles require absolute alertness, **Seldane-D**, a prescription item that contains the non-sleep-inducing antihistamine ter-fenadine along with the decongestant pseudoephedrine, would be a reasonable option.

Topical decongestants such as **Neosinephrine** nose drops or **Afrin** spray for the nasal mucosa and **Visine-Plus** for the eyes can be especially helpful for short-term use during severe attacks. Combined anti-histamine-decongestant eye drops, such as **Naphcon-A**, **Vasocon-A**, or **Opcon-A**, may need to be prescribed by your doctor.

A word of caution: Topical decongestants for either the nose or the eyes must not be used for prolonged periods of time. The immediate relief they afford often makes it tempting to continue using them beyond the three to five days recommended, but a tolerance usually develops so that you don't achieve the same degree of relief after use. But what is worse is that many people suffer a "rebound effect" in which the nasal or eye tissue actually becomes redder, sorer, and more swollen than before. In the nose, this condition, known as *rhinitis medicamentosa*, is serious and is often difficult to treat. A similar situation may result in the eyes from overuse of eye decongestants.

Treatment of rhinitis medicamentosa requires immediate cessation of the offending medication. Your doctor will probably prescribe a combination of nonmedicated saline nose sprays, such as **Ayr**, **Salinex**, or **Ocean Mist**, to soothe and lubricate the inflamed tissues of the nose, and plain **Murine** or **Visine** for the eyes, as well as a short course of topical corticosteroids to reduce the inflammation.

Other antiallergy medications include some intended to prevent allergy attacks and others for controlling severe attacks. Cromolyn sodium, found in the medications **Nasalcrom** for the nose and **Opticrom** for the eyes, has been found useful for preventing the release of histamine from mast cells. These medications are of little use for acute attacks but may be helpful if started a few weeks before the expected beginning of the allergy season. For optimal results they must be taken from four to six times per day.

For severe attacks that cannot be controlled by either antihistamines or decongestants, whether used alone or in combination, your doctor may prescribe one or more of the various corticosteroid medications currently available. Not to be confused with anabolic steroids, the sex hormone steroids abused by some body builders and athletes, corticosteroids are instead anti-inflammatory agents. Nevertheless, because they are powerful medications with a number of potential side effects, their use demands close medical supervision. They may be administered orally (such as prednisone), by injection, or as nasal sprays (such as **Vancenase**, **Beconase**, and **Nasalide**) and eye drops (such as **Decadron**).

Lastly, if you are medically unable to use conventional allergy medications or if other forms of therapy have not proven successful, your doctor may suggest allergy shots. In brief, the principle behind this form of treatment is the stimulation of IgG antibodies in response to the injection of increasingly potent doses of an allergen usually administered once or twice weekly for several months before the onset of the allergy season. Enough IgG is generally produced in this way to effectively compete with the allergy-triggering IgE antibodies that abound during the allergy season. Unfortunately, not all people respond. But allergy shots, also called *desensitization shots*, are believed to be effective, at least to some extent, in as many as 80 to 90 percent of hay fever cases. The disadvantages of this form of therapy include the inconveniences of time, discomfort, and expense and the lack of guaranteed results. For some individuals, however, these shots provide the only consistent form of relief (either by themselves or in combination with the other therapies described above).

PREVENTING ATTACKS

Finally, a few simple environmental measures may also be helpful in reducing exposure to seasonal allergens. For example, installing an air conditioner, at least in your bedroom, may be of some benefit, although complete relief from symptoms by this means can be expected in only very mild cases. Air-conditioner filters should of course be cleaned regularly to prevent the buildup of pollen and spores. If you have central air conditioning, you might also consider installing electrostatic filters in the ducts (see Chapter 3) to trap pollens and molds. Similarly, when possible, driving with your windows closed and the air conditioner on is an effective means of reducing exposure. Open car windows may expose you to as much as fifty times the amount of pollen that would otherwise reach you.

You must be especially careful outdoors. Avoid weed patches and uncut fields as much as possible, and if you plan any gardening, use a mouth and nose mask, either a double-layer surgical mask or 3M's #1800 Dust and Pollen Filter Mask. Be sure to wash your hair and launder your clothing as soon as possible afterward, especially if you have been raking leaves or mowing grass. Better still, if possible, hire a gardener. Schedule your hunting or camping trips for off-allergy-season periods. And lastly, because alcohol intake can stimulate mucus production, keep drinking to a minimum when your symptoms are at a maximum.

Taken together, these measures are practical options for most people and are better than picking up stakes entirely and moving to some other region of the country in the hope of escaping allergies.

CHAPTER THREE

YOUR HOME MAY NOT BE YOUR CASTLE: PERENNIAL ALLERGIC RHINITIS

F or those of you who think that your problems would be over if you retreated indoors, you will be saddened to learn that your home may not truly be your castle. The air indoors is often filled with an array of potential allergens, including dust, mites, mold spores, animal dander, saliva, and dried food particles. If hay fever sufferers are sometimes said to have "allergic noses," then those unfortunate souls who have year-round allergies to these abundant allergens certainly merit the same description. And since the upper respiratory symptoms that are typically provoked persist throughout the year, these allergies are aptly referred to as perennial allergic rhinitis.

DUST

Dust is so abundant that most of us take it for granted that we know what it is. But to say that dust is merely floating "dirt" that settles on your furniture or clothing is only partly correct. While it can be glamorously described as dazzling, dancing, iridescent swirls of particles seen when a beam of sunlight shines through a window, it is more complex than that; it is a mixture of many things in the home environment. It may be an accumulation of any or all of the following: outside dust, pollens, dried food particles, mold spores, insect parts and droppings, lint, synthetic fibers, hair fragments, powders, hair spray mists, animal dander, dried saliva and urine, and shed human skin cells. In genetically predisposed individuals, any or all of the many components of dust may be allergenic. (Because the issue of perennial allergies to household pets is an important and often emotionally charged one, it will be discussed in a separate chapter.)

The contribution to allergies by whole insects or bug fragments, such as wings, and the excrement they deposit everywhere deserves a few words by itself. It is very likely that most dust contains insect fragments to some extent, and they are believed to be the sources of troublesome allergies for many people. Insects whose remains have been commonly associated with respiratory allergies include the caddis fly, mayfly, and the elm bark beetle. The airborne parts or excreta from other insects, including the house mite (discussed below), may also trigger allergies in certain people.

But the ubiquitous cockroach appears to be especially problematic. It is estimated that millions of people are allergic to them—mostly to their body parts, not the feces. In one study of one hundred asthmatics in southwest Chicago, investigators found that 60 percent of them were allergic to cockroaches or their debris and required repeated hospitalization despite the regular use of their medications.

MOLDS

In Chapter 2 you learned about the two main kinds of outdoor molds that can trigger seasonal allergic rhinitis. Indoors, three other varieties are known to cause perennial allergies: *Penicillium, Aspergillus,* and *Rhizopus.* Penicillium is the fuzzy greenish mold that you may have seen growing on refrigerator walls, and Aspergillus and Rhizopus are the dark fuzzy molds that grow on bread, onions, and spoiled foods.

But molds can grow just about anywhere in your home: on floors, carpets, walls, and bathroom tiles; on wallpaper, paint, plastic, wood, leather, cotton, wool, linen, silk, rayon; on soiled upholstery, bedding, pillows (especially foam rubber ones), flowers, waste bins, old books, and magazines; and even in humidifiers and air-conditioning systems. Some species feed on the sulfur grains in concrete; others feed on the metal in paints or the glue in wallpaper. Still others are notorious for spoiling all kinds of breads, cakes, fruits, and meat products. And because of their particular growth requirements, they prefer damp, dark basements and attics. Motels, hotels, and summer cottages that are closed up for long periods of time are ideal sites for their growth and proliferation. *Mildew*, which is usually associated with a musty odor, is the more common name for the whitish powder produced by certain household molds.

Sometimes our exposure to molds comes from sources we might not readily associate with them. For example, they are intentionally placed in certain food products by manufacturers. Aged cheeses often depend on Aspergillus and Penicillium for their distinctive flavors, and Aspergillus is also used in the production of soy sauce. And while almost everyone is aware that yeast is used in the making of breads and cakes, some may not realize its importance in the fermentation of beer and wine.

Depending on the nature of their work or hobbies, some people are at greater risk for exposure to molds and thus to the development of mold allergies. Given what has already been said, you can probably guess that those who are most likely to run into mold spore allergy problems are food and drug processors, such as bakers, wine and beer brewers, butchers, cheese handlers, farmers, and pharmaceutical workers; furniture producers, such as carpenters and mattress makers; flower and plant specialists, such as florists, gardeners, greenhouse and nursery workers, and landscapers; and fabric and paper handlers, such as mill workers, newspaper and book handlers, wallpaper hangers, and furriers. Naturally, for the individual already predisposed to mold allergies, working with any of these materials can be an allergy nightmare.

Interestingly, some individuals who demonstrate airborne sensitivity to mold spores may also develop nasal and other allergy symptoms from *consuming* moldy items. Food products most likely to trigger allergy problems are aged cheeses, fermented foods, meats, and those designed for long shelf lives. The following are examples of items that either contain molds or are likely to become mold contaminated: beer, wine, and cider; buttermilk, sour cream, and cheeses; breads and cakes; beets, canned tomatoes, and mushrooms; dried fruits; smoked or pickled fish and meats; ketchup, pickles, olives, relishes, sauerkraut, salad dressings, and vinegary foods.

HOUSE MITES

Whether you like it or not, your home, no matter how clean you keep it, is filled with all kinds of bugs. But from an allergy perspective, the most troublesome by far are house mites.

House mites are tiny eight-legged creatures belonging to the *arachnid* class of organisms, which are distantly related to the spider. Two kinds of mites, *Dermatophagoides pteronyssinus* and *Dermatophagoides farinae*, are the major culprits in mite-related allergic rhinitis. Either or both of these organisms may be present in the home and responsible for the symptoms. The average amount of humidity, 60 percent, and the average temperature, 70 degrees, found year-round in most climate-controlled homes are ideal conditions for the proliferation of these bugs. In general, they abound in the East and in the Gulf Coast areas of the United States; they are seldom found in the Rocky Mountain states due to the less favorable climatic conditions for them in those regions.

The name *Dermatophagoides* means "eats skin"; it is an appropriate name for these tiny creatures because they feed primarily on skin cells shed from humans and pets and on feather-stuffed bedding and furniture. Since skin cells literally cascade off by the tens of thousands each minute whenever you walk, move around on furniture or bedding, or brush off your clothing, the hungry mites in your home do not have far to go for their next meal.

Interestingly, "so-called" allergies to feathers are seldom allergies to the feathers themselves; instead, they are reactions to the house mites that live among and feed on the feathers, which are very closely related chemically to skin cells. This means that rather than just avoiding bird feathers, you should be very cautious around down pillows, comforters, quilts, sleeping bags, and jackets because of their high mite concentrations. And the older the product, the more likely that it will cause problems due to a high concentration of mites.

Not surprisingly, the greatest number of house mites are found in and around areas where humans and pets spend most of their time—loose, long-pile carpeting, upholstered furniture, stuffed toys, clothing, and bedding. It has been estimated that forty-two thousand mites are in each ounce of mattress dust, making a grand total of about two million mites in the average double bed. In addition, each mite produces ten airborne pellets of feces each day, magnifying the overall house dust problem.

Products containing kapok, a cottony fiber derived from the fruit of the silk cotton tree found in Central and South America, may also provoke attacks of perennial allergic rhinitis in some predisposed people. Dry, lightweight, and buoyant, kapok is used to stuff mattresses, pillows, sleeping bags, and life vests. It is also found in carpet padding, upholstered furniture, and the linings of some heavy coats. As in the case of feathers, allergic reactions to the material are believed to be related to the invasion of house dust mites rather than to the fibers themselves. Once again, the older the item, the more troublesome it is likely to be.

DIAGNOSING
PERENNIAL ALLERGIC RHINITIS

The signs and symptoms of perennial allergic rhinitis are essentially the same as those for their seasonal counterparts. These include the itchy, runny, and stopped-up noses typical of rhinitis and episodic bouts of sneezing. The most notable difference between seasonal and perennial allergies, however, is that the symptoms of the latter are worse indoors; the misery persists with little abatement throughout the entire year. This means that people who suffer with allergy symptoms during the midsummer or late autumn and winter when pollen counts tend to be low are more likely to be suffering indoor mold and house dust allergies than pollen allergies. Finally, early morning and nighttime fits of sneezing are other useful clues to indoor mold and dust problems.

You should of course see your doctor to confirm that you are suffering with a perennial allergy rather than with some other condition that masquerades as one. As with seasonal allergic rhinitis, allergists can perform both blood and skin tests for a variety of potential mold, dust, mite, and insect allergens to determine what specifically triggers your problem.

COPING WITH PERENNIAL ALLERGIC RHINITIS

Because so much depends on the genes inherited by the individual and because doctors are not yet able to perform the necessary genetic manipulations to bring about complete cures, measures to prevent or minimize exposure become critical steps in the management of all patients with allergies. Few would disagree when it comes to allergies that an ounce of prevention is worth a ton of cure.

Mold-proofing Your Home

Keeping indoor mold counts down means finding all damp, poorly lit, and poorly ventilated places in your home. Like many other fungi, molds thrive in dark, damp areas where there is little circulation of air. As a result, eliminating molds requires that you find the trouble spots and reverse each of the three factors that promote mold proliferation.

In your mold hunt, pay particular attention to attics, crawl spaces, basements, laundry rooms, bathrooms, and kitchens. Air that is moving and cooler holds less moisture, so an air conditioner or fan would be advisable for the basement, kitchen, and especially the bedrooms. Damp houses may be dried by turning up the heat for a time and then opening the windows to let out the moisture-laden air. The installation and use of an exhaust fan can be especially helpful for this. Dust-collecting furniture, books, carpets, bedding, wallpaper, blinds, drapes, and so forth, should be cleaned and aired thoroughly. Bathroom and kitchen tiles, toilets, tubs, shower stalls and curtains, walls, and floors should be cleaned and dried. Because it makes a great hideout for molds, examine wallpaper, especially behind furniture. The underside of porches and the insides of closets are other trouble spots that should be cleaned thoroughly. For all of these purposes, a household chlorine bleach such as Clorox makes an effective antimildew cleanser. Lysol, a well-known commercial disinfectant, also works quite well. Wherever possible, choose mold-inhibiting paints for areas that tend to get damp.

Pillows, mattresses, and box springs, particularly their undersides, should be aired thoroughly before use and covered with impermeable plastic, vinyl, or canvas. (Sturdy airtight coverings capable of withstanding multiple washings may be ordered from Allergen-Proof Encasings, Inc., P.O. Box 5236, 1450 East 363rd Street, East Lake, Ohio 44094.) Foam rubber and urethane, while generally nonproblematic in themselves, should nonetheless be avoided because their porous construction allows for the quick accumulation of dust and mites.

Finally, before storing, make sure that all clothing, shoes, boots, and so forth, are thoroughly cleaned and dried. Even minute amounts of grease on these items makes a wonderful medium for the growth of molds.

By lessening humidity and circulating and filtering the air, air conditioners make excellent additions to antiallergy-proofing rooms. But if they are not cleaned regularly and thoroughly, particularly the filters, they may make the problem worse. To destroy another potential breeding ground for molds, you might consider periodically dropping a chlorine tablet into the place where the water drains from your window unit. For the same reasons, don't forget to routinely clean the filters in your home heating unit.

Since the average household releases as much as two quarts of water a day into the air from cooking, bathing, showering, and laundering clothes, the use of a mechanical dehumidifier to reduce dampness can be extremely helpful, especially in basements. These units should be set to maintain a uniform household humidity of 40 percent. To prevent a buildup of molds and other germs, you must clean dehumidifiers regularly.

Humidifiers, vaporizers, and steam inhalators, which are sometimes used to unclog stuffy noses, should be avoided entirely. In addition to adding moisture, they are well-known to disperse mold and bacteria into the air. Ultrasonic humidifiers, however, which employ high-frequency vibrations to convert water into mist, do not appear to increase mold and germ problems when distilled water is used and they are cleaned daily. If tap water is substituted for distilled water, which many people do to save time and money, microscopic particles of irritating minerals contained in the water may be dispersed into the air and may trigger a variety of respiratory irritations.

Finally, if possible, you should install air filters in your home's ventilation system. Two main types of filters are available: mechanical and electrostatic. As the name suggests, mechanical filters physically trap particles of dust, pollen, molds, and dander and can be extremely effective in removing possible allergens. In fact, when a HEPA (High Efficiency Particulate Accumulator) filter is used in a central system, virtually 99 percent of home air pollutants may be eliminated. These filters are composed of an interwoven network of tiny glass fibers that are capable of trapping minute particles.

Electrostatic filters work by a different method. First they cause dust and other unwanted particles to become negatively charged, and then they capture the particles as they pass oppositely charged wires in the system. Electrostatic filters are generally effective in central systems, but they must be cleaned frequently to maintain optimal functioning. Some of these units have been associated with the emission of small amounts of ozone, which may be irritating to the mucous membranes of the eyes and the respiratory system.

If you do not have a central air system, freestanding filters are also available for use in single rooms. For best results you should choose a HEPA-containing unit, one that is large enough to turn over air in the room many times per hour. An ordinary unit capable of adequately filtering a bedroom would be about the size of a night table. Desktop units are usually too small to do an adequate job. (And when prescribed by your doctor, the installation of air filters may be tax deductible.)

Dust and Mite-proofing the House

Unfortunately, no matter how meticulous you are, it is impossible to totally remove all dust from your house. Nevertheless, every attempt should be made to reduce the dust content as much as possible. And the room that should receive your most intense efforts is the bedroom, where you spend an average of eight hours out of twenty-four—nearly one-third of your life. For most of us, the family room or den would be next on the list. If you feel unusually energetic, you can continue on, possibly attempting to reduce dust throughout the entire house.

Doing the job right is no small task. First you must remove all the furnishings from the room. Everything! Clear out the furniture, the beds, the draperies, and the curtains. Empty out the closets and remove the books, bookcases, knickknacks, and bric-a-brac. Remove any area rugs and, if possible, get rid of all carpeting. Recent evidence suggests that this is probably the single most important step for reducing house mites because these items are their main nesting areas.

Next, if possible, have a nonallergic relative or friend clean all the removed items *outside* the room. The last thing you want is to have all that dust spewed into the air by cleaning things in the room. Since dry dusting and sweeping only make things worse by whipping the dust into the air where it can remain suspended for hours, the walls and ceiling of the room should be damp-dusted and the floors damp-mopped.

Afterward, look over all the furnishings and select only the items that are absolutely essential to you. In general, you would do well to restrict your bedroom to a bed, chair, night table, and chest of drawers. The fewer the pieces, the better. Dust collectors such as books, knickknacks, picture frames, and lamp shades should be removed, and storage items should be placed elsewhere. And because they are more easily cared for and cleaned, choose wooden, plastic, or metal pieces rather than use upholstered fabrics. Replace all feather pillows and comforters with those made from Dacron or polyester. Store all regularly used clothing in vinyl zippered clothing bags. Use easily washable 100 percent cotton or plastic curtains, avoid draperies and venetian blinds, and opt for a plain wooden or linoleum-covered floor rather than carpets or rugs.

If you simply must have some kind of flooring, purchase short-nap, washable synthetics or 100 percent cotton rugs and use only synthetic underpadding or, better, none at all. But if you cannot bear to part with your carpet, you may try treating it with Allergy Control Solution, which contains 3 percent tannic acid. Tannic acid, the main ingredient in tea, has been found to inactivate the allergy-provoking effects of mite allergens. One treatment may be effective for up to two months. Alternatively, the carpet may be periodically sprayed with Acarosan, which contains the antimite chemical benzyl benzoate, or with RID spray, which contains pyrethrin. The effects of these agents may also remain for several months.

Cleaning your allergy-proofed room once a week should become routine. More frequent cleaning is not suggested, however, because it is likely to stir up dust; it is generally better to do fewer, more thorough cleanings than more frequent, less diligent ones. Be sure to clean the furniture and wall surfaces with a damp cloth, and the floors and ceilings with a damp mop. Curtains should also be washed weekly and are best left either open or closed all the time so as not to scatter dust when moving them. Although convenient, vacuum cleaners are actually ill-advised since they are often responsible for scattering millions of microscopic dust particles, either through the exhaust or by escape through the bag itself.

Finally, don't forget the bedding in your once-a-week cleaning. Use *hot* water when laundering since house mites generally survive cold water washing.

Finally, as in the case of reducing mold exposure, the use of air filters can be extremely helpful.

MEDICAL TREATMENTS

As in the case of seasonal allergic rhinitis, antihistamines and decongestants are the mainstays of therapy for all forms of perennial allergic rhinitis. For some people allergy shots (desensitization) may also be effective, especially when combined with the preventive measures described above.

CHAPTER FOUR

WHEN FIDO GIVES YOU MORE THAN JUST LOVE: COPING WITH PET ALLERGIES

J ust about everyone has heard something about allergies to pets. Unfortunately, many of those sweet, lovable, huggable, and kissable "family members," including "man's best friend," are all too often one of the causes of the miseries of perennial allergic rhinitis, the so-called allergic nose. It has been estimated that as much as 10 percent of the population is at risk of developing pet allergies and that between 15 percent and 30 percent of all allergy-prone individuals may be allergic to cats and dogs. Considering that more than 100 million pet dogs and cats are in more than half of the homes in the United States, the problem of pet allergies is not a small one. And these figures do not include the countless guinea pigs, hamsters, mice, rats, rabbits, and birds that are also kept as pets both at home and in schools.

Since our pets obviously mean so much to us, the issue of possible allergies to them is often an emotionally charged one for many allergy sufferers. And while these allergies technically have much in common with respiratory allergies to dust, molds, and mites, the unwillingness of many loyal pet owners to part with Fido or Samantha despite the misery of their symptoms makes allergies to pets worthy of discussion on its own.

WHAT CAUSES PET ALLERGIES?

Contrary to conventional wisdom, animal hairs are *not* the real culprits in the overwhelming majority of pet allergies. In the first place, the proteins in hair are not particularly allergenic. In the second place, because hairs are relatively large and heavy materials that tend to settle where they fall, they do not ordinarily remain airborne long enough to trigger significant allergic respiratory problems. Obviously, then, there is little merit to the widely held belief that long-haired breeds are more allergy-provoking than short-haired ones.

If your pet's hairs are not the real problem, then what is? The answer is that animal dander, the flaky, dandrufflike skin cells that your pet sheds by the millions each day, is believed to be the chief allergy troublemaker. Like pollens and mold spores, dander is considered an *aeroallergen* because it can be easily blown about by the air and is small enough to remain airborne for many hours. As a result, dander may be inhaled deeply into the breathing tubes and lungs where it is capable of producing severe allergic reactions. Individuals with a family or personal history of asthma, hay fever, or eczema appear to be especially prone to pet allergies.

But dander is not the only culprit that has been linked to pet allergies. Pets also shed other kinds of allergens into the air, mostly from their saliva and urine. When these fluids dry out on carpets or furniture surfaces, they then can flake off, become airborne, and eventually permeate the entire house. In general, these substances are sticky and attach to walls, clothing, and even other dust particles. In this way they are spread over large areas, causing problems throughout the home—and even in homes that have never had pets.

DOG ALLERGIES

Although some allergy sufferers swear that they are allergic to one breed of dog and not another, there is little hard medical evidence to support it. What may account for that misconception is that some breeds shed more allergenic materials than others from their skin and saliva, while others produce a greater volume of saliva or skin cells. Nonetheless, the basic dog allergens responsible for provoking allergic symptoms are essentially the same from one breed to the next. This means that prolonged contact with dogs of any breed will eventually trigger allergy symptoms in susceptible individuals.

Confusion may arise when a dog owner who is accustomed to the ebb and flow of low-grade symptoms at home visits a neighbor and experiences a dramatic flare-up of his allergy when exposed to the neighbor's dog. The response is usually to blame the neighbor's dog erroneously and attribute the allergy to that specific breed. In actuality, the onset of the attack was the result of a more intense exposure to dog allergen at the neighbor's house rather than exposure to an altogether new kind of allergen.

CAT ALLERGIES

With no intention of offending any feline admirers, pet cats as a rule trigger more allergic reactions than their canine counterparts. This is attributable to the fact that cats tend to be more fastidious in their personal hygiene, and lick and groom themselves more often. While this may be a source of pride for pet owners, it also means that more potentially allergenic cat saliva allergens are spewed into the air they breathe. As in the case of dogs, all breeds of cats, regardless of the length of their fur, are about the same in their ability to provoke allergic reactions in humans.

ALLERGIES TO OTHER PETS

After cats and dogs, sportsmen should be aware that horses are the next most common cause of animal allergies. But in the home, other family favorites such as birds, gerbils, guinea pigs, hamsters, mice, rats, and rabbits may also be a source of perennial allergies. In each of these cases, dander and especially substances in the urine and saliva are once again believed to be more important allergens than either fur or feathers. In most cases allergies to feathers are really allergies to the mites that live within them and not to the feathers themselves.

Unfortunately, even when a pet owner is willing to trade in his favorite furry companion for the sake of his allergies (which few are usually willing to do), the solution may not lie in simply substituting one kind of pet for another because allergy-prone people are usually allergic to more than one kind of pet. For example, it is estimated that somewhere between 20 percent and 40 percent of allergic people possess allergies to *both* dogs and cats. It is also believed that after prolonged exposure, between 40 percent and 60 percent of these same individuals would also develop allergies to guinea pigs and hamsters. If you are contemplating any exchanges, hairless creatures would be your best bet. In general, tropical fish, turtles, hermit crabs, and snakes do not provoke allergies and therefore make safe alternatives for allergy sufferers.

COTTONSEED OIL AND LINSEED

Cottonseed oil and linseed are two possible sources of pet-related allergy that deserve special note. Cottonseed meal is a highly allergenic material found in certain kinds of baked goods (such as buns, brown cookies, glazed doughnuts, and fried cakes), pan-greasing compounds, and salad oils. But most important for the purposes of this discussion, it is also found in certain animal foods. For some people, exposure to dust from this material can trigger severe debilitating allergy symptoms. In this event the allergy is clearly not directly related to your pet but to what your pet eats. This is an eminently easier problem to remedy because you can change the animal's diet. (Note: The cottonseed oil found in Spry, Crisco, and Wesson oils is highly processed and is generally not considered to be allergenic.)

Linseed, or flaxseed, is found in a number of common products including some depilatories, insulation, carpeting materials, hair-waving preparations, and shampoos. It may also be inhaled from cattle and poultry feed and dog food. For some individuals, especially asthmatics, linseed can be extremely irritating and may even provoke severe attacks. Once again, changing the animal's food may be all that it is needed to reduce symptoms.

DIAGNOSING PET ALLERGIES

The miseries experienced because of pet allergies—that is, the itchy eyes, fits of sneezing, runny nose, and stuffy head of dust and indoor mold allergies—are virtually indistinguishable from the signs and symptoms of other perennial allergies. Although less common than respiratory difficulties, hives are another well-recognized manifestation of an allergy to pets. They frequently occur as a result of direct contact with pet allergens. For example, they may break out when allergens get on the hands from petting the pet or touching other contaminated surfaces, or in places where the animal has licked the skin or a rough tail has abraded it.

To determine whether Fido is the cause of your problems or just the scapegoat, your doctor may recommend allergy testing. This usually involves skin tests or a specialized blood examination known as the RAST (see Appendix A). It is understandable when pet owners continue to deny emphatically that their pet is the root of their suffering, even when they are faced with the corroborating evidence of lab tests. A trial separation for the pet and the pet owner of several weeks might fail to prove to the owner that the pet is at fault because it can take several months before household levels of pet allergens fall to levels that they no longer provoke significant allergy symptoms. Moreover, some pet owners become so accustomed to their symptoms at home that they recognize a worsening only when they visit the home of someone else who owns a pet; this can make the allergy link to their own pet all the more improbable to them.

WHAT TO DO

The logical treatment for a proven pet allergy is to give away the pet. Since this is an unacceptable solution for many people, some commonsense measures can prove very helpful for reducing symptoms even if Fido stays.

The first thing you can do is keep your pet out of the bedroom. Since most people spend the majority of their time at home in the bedroom, it makes good sense to banish your pet from that room in order to reduce your exposure to allergens. It has been estimated that doing so will result in a thousandfold decrease in exposure. The same logic applies to any other room in the house where you spend a good deal of your time, such as a study.

Once you have placed your bedroom off-limits, you should also remove all contaminated carpeting and bedding; these items are chock-full of allergens and can remain so long after your pet has been exiled from the room. A simple cleaning or vacuuming is not recommended, however. For one thing, not enough allergens are removed that way, and for another, you may make matters worse by stirring things up and spewing more allergens into the air. If you can, it is best to replace all fabrics and carpets with brand-new ones. Room air cleaners, either the electrostatic variety or the HEPA (High Efficiency Particulate Accumulator) filters, may also be useful. Finally, a word of warning is in order: If you relent, even once, and let your pet back into the room, you may defeat all your good, hard work.

There is one useful preventive measure that unfortunately runs contrary to environmental protection and energy efficiency recommendations, namely, deinsulating your home. Well-insulated homes may contain as much as five times the amount of pet allergens as their more poorly insulated counterparts, even when such homes use HEPA filters on the furnaces. If you are lucky enough to have a backyard, however, you can let your pet roam outside as much as possible when you are at home (weather permitting, of course). And if weather conditions in your area are moderate for a good part of the year, you may even consider building separate living quarters for your pooch outdoors. This will also lower your exposure to allergens.

Another important measure is to bathe your pet frequently. This rids the fur of allergens as well as other possible troublemakers such as pollens. Bathing has recently been found to be particularly important in dealing with cat allergies. One of the most important allergens produced by cats is a sticky protein substance known as Fel dI, which is secreted by their oil glands. Monthly bathing has been found to reduce and in many cases entirely halt production of this protein.

The cleaning routine is fairly simple, and after only one or two times, most cats become quite used to it, especially if you start them when they are kittens. Begin by placing your cat in a basin of warm water. Next, slowly pour plain tap water (or distilled water, if you prefer) over your pet; rub the fur gently as you pour the water. Be especially careful to avoid getting it into the animal's eyes and ears. You may prefer to use cotton balls to protect the ears. For optimal results, you must repeat the cleaning procedure several times. When you have finished, press as much of the water from the fur as possible (it contains the Fel dI), and then towel-dry thoroughly. Do not blow-dry! Performing this procedure monthly for several months will result in a dramatic decrease or complete cessation of allergen production (spelling relief from your symptoms) and will in no way harm your pet.

Regular brushing and grooming is another important measure. It almost goes without saying that the pet should not be brushed indoors, and if you are the allergic one in the family, have someone else do the brushing, if possible. When that is not possible, you may find air filter masks and protective clothing helpful for reducing exposure. And if your clothing becomes contaminated by contact with the pet, change as soon as possible and launder thoroughly. This is also good advice following a visit to a neighbor's home where there is a pet.

THERAPY

The mainstays of therapy are similar to those used to treat other causes of perennial allergic rhinitis such as dust, mite, and mold allergies. Treatments include the use of a wide variety of antihistamines, nasal and oral corticosteroid drugs, and cromolyn sodium. When all else fails, short of getting rid of your beloved pet, you may consider allergy shots or immunotherapy (see Appendix B). Some recent studies have indicated that these shots, while more effective if initiated before exposure to a pet, may be helpful in reducing the severity of symptoms. To date they have proven of the greatest value in lessening flare-ups in individuals who are subject to occasional unavoidable social contact with pets. Nevertheless, they are certainly worth exploring when Fido is too lovable to part with and animal allergen exposure cannot be otherwise effectively reduced.

CHAPTER FIVE

WHEN AN ALLERGY IS NOT JUST SOMETHING TO SNEEZE AT: ASTHMA

A sthma is one condition that should never be confused with simple allergy. Triggered or aggravated by a variety of irritants and allergens, it is a complex disorder affecting the large and small breathing tubes leading to the lungs. And while the stuffy head, watery eyes, runny nose, and fits of sneezing so typical of seasonal and perennial allergies may occasionally make you feel as though you are dying, the far more serious respiratory condition of asthma can be truly life-threatening in some instances.

According to the National Institute of Allergy and Infectious Diseases, asthma, or bronchial asthma as it is sometimes called, represents a staggering public health problem. It has been estimated that between ten and twelve million people in the United States alone suffer from some form of this condition. This translates into more than 1.8 million emergency room interventions, twenty-seven million outpatient visits, and nearly half a million hospitalizations annually. Because of it, workers lose millions of workdays, countless others must go on permanent disability, and children between the ages of six and fifteen miss more than 125 million days of school every year.

The economic consequences may be equally devastating. Victims annually spend over $300 million for needed ongoing evaluation and treatment and more than $1 billion for medications. It is estimated that these expenditures consume nearly a fifth of the entire family income of the average asthma sufferer. Unfortunately, since it is anticipated that the number of newly diagnosed cases of asthma will continue to rise, we can reasonably expect these statistics to worsen.

WHAT IS ASTHMA?

Asthma is by no means a new medical condition. Over two thousand years ago, it was already well known to the ancient Greeks who gave it its present name, which aptly means "to breathe hard." In the simplest terms, asthma is a breathing disorder, but in order to understand what happens during a typical asthma attack, you need to know some basics about the process of breathing and the anatomy of the respiratory system.

Under normal circumstances, when you breathe, air is drawn in through your mouth and nose and enters the chest through a large tube known as the *trachea*, or windpipe. At its base the windpipe divides into two slightly smaller, muscular breathing tubes known as the *bronchi* (singular: *bronchus*). The bronchus that leads to the right lung is called the *right bronchus*, and the one to the left lung is the *left bronchus*. Each bronchus further divides and subdivides within the lungs to form hundreds of microscopic breathing tubes called *bronchioles*, and thousands of air sacs, called *alveoli*. It is through the thin walls of these air sacs that inhaled oxygen is transferred to the blood and carbon dioxide and other waste gases are discharged from the body when exhaled through your nose and mouth.

The healthy respiratory system possesses several efficient means of ridding itself of potential airborne troublemakers. Of these, mucus and cilia are perhaps the two most important cleansing and eliminating mechanisms. Mucus, secreted by special cells called *goblet cells* that line the breathing tubes, serves as the chief cleaning and lubricating fluid of the respiratory system. *Cilia*, which are the many thousands of tiny, beating hairlike fibers that line the tubes, continually drive mucus and other debris upward toward the mouth and nose where they may be easily eliminated.

Asthma attacks can be thought of as a disruption in the delicate workings of the breathing system, and these attacks involve three events: spasm, swelling, and excessive mucus production. *Bronchospasm* occurs early in an attack. This is a response to inhaled germs, irritants, or allergens in which the muscle fibers making up the walls of the bronchi contract involuntarily and forcefully. It is believed to result from dysfunction of the autonomic nervous system, that branch of your nervous system over which you have no conscious control. *Airway hyperreactivity*, a term often used by doctors, is another name for bronchospasm.

At about the same time in the an asthma attack, the mucus-producing cells lining the breathing tubes begin producing large amounts of thick, sticky, irritating mucus, or *phlegm*. Phlegm is largely responsible for triggering the coughing so characteristic of asthma.

If an attack is not checked, the walls of the bronchi soon swell from inflammation, resulting in additional narrowing or obstruction of the airways. When this occurs, excessive amounts of air eventually become trapped in the lungs, and the chest cavity swells. Attempting to exhale this increased volume of air forcibly through the markedly narrowed breathing tubes results in the wheezing characteristic of asthma. Without prompt treatment, some breathing tubes plug with mucus and others close off entirely, causing shortness of breath, a feeling of gasping for air, and speechlessness. Prompt intervention generally restores breathing to normal, and for that reason asthma is defined as an "intermittent, reversible, obstructive airway disease."

Signs and Symptoms

Coughing, wheezing, and shortness of breath are characteristic of asthma. Caused by either the mucus buildup or the spasm in the airways, the cough may be either full and loose, or dry and hacking. Like most asthma symptoms, the severity of coughing may vary during an attack—tending to be milder early on and progressively more debilitating later. When an attack is over and the narrowed airways start reopening, sufferers may occasionally find themselves coughing up tiny tube-shaped mucus plugs.

Wheezing is perhaps the hallmark of asthma, plaguing virtually all asthmatics. A wheeze is the sound created by air when it is forced through abnormally narrowed breathing tubes. Wheezing can fluctuate from mild to severe during an attack and may be heard on both inhaling and exhaling. Curiously, some asthmatics become so accustomed to their own chronic wheezing that they hardly notice it until they perform some activity that raises their usual, baseline rate of breathing.

Finally, shortness of breath, or *dyspnea*, is another characteristic asthma symptom. When severe, it may be accompanied by profuse sweating and a panicky feeling of choking or gasping for air.

The time it takes for a severe asthma attack to develop varies and is generally unpredictable. Sometimes it takes hours and other times days. But no matter how long it takes, the overall course is typified by a relentless worsening of symptoms. For this reason it is important to become familiar with your own pattern of symptoms so that therapy may be initiated early—when the airway problems are more easily reversible. For those with a history of severe attacks, prompt medical attention may be crucial.

WHO GETS IT

Asthma tends to run in families, and the fact that many asthmatics have relatives with the problem lends strong weight to the notion of an inherited (or genetic) basis for the disorder. If one parent has it, there is a 25 percent chance that his or her offspring will also have it. When both parents do, the chance of the child having it climbs to 50 percent.

Asthma may make its first appearance at any age. While it frequently begins during infancy, it has also been known to strike without prior warning around the time of menopause. In childhood, the majority of sufferers experience their first symptoms sometime before the first grade. In general, for any age range in the United States, more males are affected than females.

WHAT CAUSES IT

Not all cases of asthma are triggered by allergies. When it is, the condition is described as *extrinsic* asthma, or asthma arising from an outside cause. When allergies do not appear to play a role, the condition is known as *intrinsic* asthma, meaning that it stems from factors within the individual. Most cases of asthma are not so clear-cut, however; they may result from a combination of both allergic and nonallergic factors. Nevertheless, one thing that asthma is not is contagious. In other words, you cannot give your asthma to your friends or contract it from anyone else.

Allergic (Extrinsic) Asthma

Allergic asthma tends to be triggered by the same kinds of allergens as those known to provoke seasonal and perennial allergic rhinitis, namely dust, dander, molds, and pollens. Certain food additives (such as metabisulfites and monosodium glutamate [MSG]), industrial and occupational chemicals, and a number of medications (aspirin, for example) have also been linked to asthma in some cases. Regardless of the allergen, the allergic events that lead to asthma, after exposure to a particular allergen, share much in common with what occurs in, say, pollen allergies. One major distinction, however, is that asthma affects the lower breathing tubes and the lungs, while seasonal and perennial allergies primarily involve the nasal passages and sinuses.

Nonallergic (Intrinsic) Asthma

Although our concern is with allergic conditions, no discussion of asthma would be complete without describing the various nonallergic triggers of the disorder. These include stress, exercise, sex, upper gastrointestinal problems, upper respiratory virus infections, and pollutants.

Years ago many people contended that asthma was a psychosomatic disorder, the product of "nerves." Today we know that it is not a condition that is "just in the head." At the same time, stress does play a role. Many asthmatics steadfastly maintain that their symptoms are triggered or aggravated by episodes of increased nervous tension, frustration, or anger.

Experts theorize that the rapid and shallow breathing pattern (hyperventilation) that characterizes anxiety problems may be responsible for promoting bronchospasm in asthma-prone individuals. It has likewise been proposed that the alterations in this pattern brought about by biofeedback and behavior modification techniques, such as meditation and deep breathing exercises, may account for the benefits sometimes obtained from these modalities. But whatever the success of these measures, there is no scientific support for the notion that asthma is directly caused by emotional stress. What we can say for sure is that the condition itself has been the cause of a good deal of stress.

Exercise is another important factor in many asthmatics, acting as a trigger. The phenomenon is referred to as exercise-induced bronchospasm (EIB) or exercise-induced asthma (EIA). Attacks typically begin between five and ten minutes after the start of a workout. During exercise your lungs work harder, and you breathe in and out more rapidly. As a consequence the inspired and expired air becomes drier, cooler, more irritating, and more likely to precipitate an asthma attack in a susceptible person. It remains unclear whether it is the dryness, the coolness, or a combination of these factors that is responsible for triggering the attack. Nevertheless, in response the respiratory system releases the same kinds of mediators as seen in true allergic reactions.

Since exercise-induced attacks do not begin immediately, those sports that require only short bursts of energy rather than constant activity are generally better tolerated by most asthmatics. These include baseball, bowling, golf, lightweight training, tennis (especially doubles), and sprinting. Although swimming requires more constant activity and is generally more demanding on the respiratory system, its untoward effects appear to be offset by the moistened air that is inhaled.

Sex is another physical activity that may aggravate asthma. Even mild asthmatics may notice an increase in wheezing during lovemaking. A history of sex-related asthma may be the first clue to the physician that a patient suffers from a previously ignored mild case of the condition. Fortunately, sex-induced asthma generally responds quite well to various medications, particularly sprays, and need not be an impediment to romance.

Problems in the upper gastrointestinal system, especially hiatal hernias, may also trigger asthma attacks. Regurgitation of the stomach contents back into the esophagus, a process doctors call *gastroesophageal reflux* and that often occurs at night when the individual with a hiatus hernia is recumbent in bed, can precipitate a severe attack. Coughing can be fitful in these cases. Older individuals with hiatus hernias are especially prone. Investigators believe that in asthmatics the reflux within the gastrointestinal system sets off a reflex in the respiratory system, leading to an attack. Naturally, the gastrointestinal problem must be dealt with if the asthma is to improve.

Nocturnal asthma, another form of acute asthma that, as its name suggests, begins in the middle of the night, is unrelated to reflux but is a particular problem for a small percentage of asthmatics. Current thinking suggests that attacks are the result of the effects of normal hormonal fluctuations on asthmatic airways, and several explanations have been given for this phenomenon. For one thing, the body's natural levels of epinephrine and cortisol, two important asthma-controlling agents, are ordinarily at their lowest levels during the night; at the same time, histamine, which can worsen asthma, is at its highest level. Other explanations for nocturnal asthma include the effects of the body temperature drop that ordinarily occurs during the night, as well as the physiologic nighttime increase in the activity of the vagus nerve, which is responsible for airway constriction known as bronchostriction.

Viral respiratory infections are troublemakers for everyone, but they are especially worrisome for asthmatics, who tend also to be more susceptible to them. The increased inflammation, swelling, and thickened mucus production that these infections cause add to the already overburdened respiratory apparatus of the sufferer. The common cold, the flu, and sinus infections are particular problems for asthmatics; although equally problematic when present, bacterial infections are much less frequently responsible for triggering or aggravating asthma symptoms.

In young children, viral bronchiolitis and croup have actually been linked in some instances to the subsequent development of asthma. And in one large study of adult-onset asthmatics, nearly half of them attributed the start of their illness to a prior respiratory infection. Investigators speculate that these infectious processes sensitize the lining of the respiratory system with allergy-related IgE antibodies, setting the stage for future allergic asthma attacks.

Environmental irritants and pollutants are other well-known asthma aggravators. Atmospheric pollutants, such as ozone and sulfur dioxide, top the list, which also includes such common irritants as cigarette smoke, chimney fumes, gasoline vapor, and automotive exhaust.

It is perhaps less well known that strong odors of various kinds can also precipitate attacks. In this category, insecticides and roach sprays head the list, followed by ammonia-containing household cleansers. Nearly 75 percent of asthmatics point to colognes, perfumes, and fresh paint as other problem odors, and approximately a third of sufferers claim to be irritated by ordinary cooking smells.

DIAGNOSING ASTHMA

A history of coughing, wheezing, and shortness of breath is a good indication of underlying asthma. Since other respiratory conditions may cause these symptoms, your doctor might supplement your history, physical examination, and routine laboratory work with a variety of tests in order to confirm the diagnosis. These may include X rays, special blood tests, skin tests, and pulmonary function tests.

A chest X ray is extremely useful for excluding other chronic lung conditions, such as emphysema, or cystic fibrosis in children. It also serves as a baseline test against which future improvements may be measured.

RAST is a very sophisticated blood test that determines the level of IgE antibodies you possess to particular allergens. The main advantage of this test is that a small sample of blood may be used to test for many different allergens. The disadvantage is that the test has a lower success rate than the routine skin tests for allergens briefly described below. For this reason doctors would say that the RAST is *less sensitive* than skin testing, and owing to this, some skin testing is often necessary to supplement the RAST.

Skin tests are an important part of an asthma workup. They are not only useful for indicating what substances you are allergic to but the severity of your allergies as well. Scratch tests and puncture tests involve making a series of tiny scratches or punctures in the skin and then applying extracts of potential allergens; a positive result is the development of redness, swelling, or hives at the test sites. Intradermal tests, which are performed in the same fashion as the familiar PPD screening test for tuberculosis, are similar to scratch tests except that the material is injected superficially under the skin; again, redness, swelling, or hives suggests an allergy to the test substance.

Spirometry, or pulmonary function studies, may also be ordered to evaluate breathing function. Performed in the office, this testing essentially involves inhaling and exhaling through a tube that is attached to a recording machine which is capable of registering and graphing your level of respiratory function. The test measures not only how much air you are able to move in and out of your lungs but how quickly you can do it, both before and after the use of bronchodilator medications (see below). A marked improvement in your breathing function after the use of bronchodilators is a good indication of the presence of asthma, which by definition is largely a *reversible* airway problem. Spirometry is also useful, once a diagnosis has been confirmed, for evaluating the effectiveness of treatment.

Another instrument, the *peak flow meter*, is a small plastic device used by the patient at home to measure the rate of airflow out of the lungs. The test itself is quite simple to perform. The individual first inhales as deeply as possible and then blows out into the machine as rapidly as possible. Two readings are generally taken each day, once shortly after arising and then again later in the day. Since lung function in asthmatics is generally worse in the morning and improves as the day progresses, a decrease between the morning and afternoon readings signals a problem. In addition, comparing daily recordings is useful for assessing overall progress. These devices are mostly recommended for severe asthmatics who must keep a close watch on their respiratory status and response to medications.

TREATING ASTHMA

Preventive Measures

It goes without saying that if you know the particular factors that worsen your asthma, you should reduce your exposure to them as much as possible. For example, airborne irritants that are known to trigger bronchospasm, such as cigarette smoke, should be avoided. And since there is evidence that marijuana smoke may be twenty times more irritating than tobacco smoke, avoidance of this substance is especially prudent. Likewise, whenever possible, exposure to fumes from insecticides, hair sprays, deodorants, paints, and perfumes should be minimized. In this regard, the use of air conditioners, humidifiers, and air filters can be extremely helpful.

If feasible, you should also avoid those foods and medications that have been linked to asthma flare-ups. These include the food additive MSG, the infamous Chinese Restaurant Syndrome culprit, and the metabisulfites, which are common preservatives found in restaurant salads, many canned beverages and foods, fermented drinks, pickled vegetables, packaged dried fruits, and certain processed items such as potato chips.

A small percentage of asthmatic flare-ups have in the past been linked to exposure to *azo dyes*, which are coal tar derivatives used to color various foods and drugs. Tartrazine, also known as FD&C Yellow No. 5, is a well-known example. More recent studies have cast some doubt on the link between azo dye and asthma, however, and as of now, further investigation is needed.

Asthmatics must be especially wary of aspirin. As many as 10 percent of asthma suffers will experience a flare-up within thirty minutes of taking aspirin. And for reasons that are not entirely clear, those with a history of chronic sinus problems and nasal polyps are especially prone to this response. Adverse reactions may likewise be provoked by a number of aspirin-related medications, such as the nonsteroidal antiinflammatory drugs (NSAID) that are frequently prescribed for arthritis, musculoskeletal disorders, and menstrual problems. Familiar drugs in this category are, among others, **Advil**, **Motrin**, **Anaprox**, **Naprosyn**, **Nuprin**, **Butazolidin**, and **Indocin**.

Finally, if you have seasonal respiratory allergies, you would do well to seek treatment for them since the link between hay fever and the subsequent development of asthma is especially noteworthy. In fact, about 5 percent of children with hay fever go on to develop asthma, and as many as 40 percent of all hay fever sufferers are discovered by spirometry testing to have some form of asthmalike findings.

Specific Therapies

Unfortunately, only the mildest cases of asthma respond to preventive measures alone. Most require some form of medical therapy. Today, the most common forms of asthma medication include bronchodilators, sympathomimetic agents, mast cell stabilizers, and corticosteroids. The use of these therapies, either alone or in various combinations, has afforded millions of people relief from what would otherwise be a debilitating, if not life-threatening, disease.

Since constriction of the breathing tubes is one of the hallmarks of asthma, *bronchodilators*, which are medications aimed at opening up the airways, make up one of the mainstays of asthma therapy. Asthmatics appear to possess in their lungs an inadequate amount of an important chemical known as cyclic adenosine monophosphate, or CAMP for short, which is responsible for normal airway opening. Bronchodilators work by interfering with the enzyme in the lungs that normally breaks down CAMP, in this way increasing CAMP levels and promoting more normal airway passages.

Medications containing *theophylline* or its derivatives are probably the best-known types of bronchodilators, and with the availability today of short, intermediate, long, and twenty-four-hour preparations, we are fortunate that doctors can tailor the dose and frequency of these drugs to the specific needs of most patients. Those with mild cases generally profit from the shorter-acting varieties, while those with more chronic asthma may benefit from the longer-acting ones. Examples of short-acting preparations include **Aminophyllin**, **Bronkodyl**, **Slo-Phyllin**, and **Elixophyllin**. Intermediate theophyllines include theophylline SR, **Slo-Phyllin SR**, and **Theolair SR**. Long-acting preparations include **Theo-Dur** and **Slo-bid**. **Theo-24** and **Uniphyl** are two twenty-four-hour bronchodilators. Doctors often order periodic blood tests on patients who are taking these drugs to determine whether the level of theophylline in the bloodstream is within the desired therapeutic range.

Hormonelike drugs known as *sympathomimetic* agents are a second major class of antiasthma medication. These work to promote airway passage by stimulating an enzyme necessary for increasing CAMP levels. The name **Adrenalin**, or epinephrine, will be immediately recognized by anyone who has ever gone to the emergency room for treatment of a severe asthma attack. Usually given intravenously or by injection under the skin, epinephrine has literally been a blessing in emergency situations, although it is not for day-to-day use.

When reading about sympathomimetics in product literature or package inserts, you may come across the term *selective beta-2 activity*. All this means is that the drug has been formulated to work specifically where it is needed on certain chemical sites, known as the beta-2 receptors, located within the smooth muscles of the airways. Nonselective medications, by contrast, may affect all beta receptor sites in the body, including those within the heart where they may be responsible for such unwanted side effects as elevated blood pressure and heart rhythm abnormalities. Happily, a wide variety of selective sympathomimetic agents have been developed for daily use and are available by prescription in tablet, syrup, nebulizer (a machine that converts a liquid to a mist), or spray formulations.

Inhaled bronchodilators must be used properly to ensure maximum benefits. Most come as *metered dose inhalers*, which are hand-held, pocket-sized canisters that deliver the medication via the mouth directly into the breathing tubes. For optimal effect you need to get most of the medication deep into the lungs. In order to do this, you should keep the canister about two inches from your mouth rather than closing your lips around the mouthpiece, which is the natural tendency. By doing so, larger droplets from the inhaler are given a long enough distance to travel so that they break up into smaller droplets, which are better able to penetrate the narrower, more deeply situated branches of the breathing tubes. Alternatively, you may purchase a *spacer* device, a small tubular attachment for the inhaler that provides the optimal spacing for droplet breakup. Whatever the method of aerosol delivery, you must inhale the medication for three to five seconds and then hold your breath for up to ten seconds. Those with exercise-induced asthma might receive greater benefit by administering their dose about fifteen to twenty minutes *before* planned workouts.

Doctors usually take the patient's age and the severity of the condition into consideration when choosing the form and dosage of medication. Many specialists prefer metered dose sprays because the right amount gets to precisely where it is needed the most and with a minimum of side effects. Syrups are usually reserved for young children and adults who are unable to swallow pills. Nebulizers are used for very young children or the very elderly who are unable to manage sprays. **Proventil**, **Ventolin**, **Brethine**, **Bricanyl**, **Alupent**, and **Metaprel** are commonly prescribed forms of beta-2 sympathomimetic agents.

Many physicians advise against the use of over-the-counter, fixed drug combinations of theophyllines and sympathomimetics, such as **Primatene "P,"** **Tedral**, and **Marax**. For one thing, many of them contain the sympathomimetic agent ephedrine, which is not a selective beta-2 agent and therefore unnecessarily affects the heart. A second, no less important reason is that such combinations do not permit the flexibility of dose adjustment of the individual ingredients to meet the specific needs of an asthma sufferer. This means, for example, that a person may get too much or too little of different components. In addition, combination products may contain unnecessary ingredients. They often contain, for example, phenobarbital and antihistamines, additives that contribute little to their overall effectiveness while they increase the likelihood of adverse reactions.

Anticholinergics are another class of bronchodilators worthy of mention. These agents work by blocking the effects of the hormone-like agent *acetylcholine* on the airways. Normally secreted by the vagus nerves of the lungs, acetylcholine is responsible for increasing airway constriction and mucus production. Anticholinergics, such as the **Atrovent** inhaler, have been found to be very useful for maintenance therapy rather than for acute treatment.

Cromolyn sodium (for example, **Intal**) is another very important drug in your doctor's antiasthma armamentarium. Neither a theophylline nor a sympathomimetic, the drug is believed to work by several important mechanisms. Most important, it blocks mast cell release of histamine, thereby reducing inflammation and alleviating any underlying allergic components of the asthma. Through an indirect mechanism, it may also raise CAMP levels and reduce bronchospasm. Finally, it is believed to possess a separate, direct antiinflammatory action that is capable of further reducing tissue swelling and sensitivity. In general, cromolyns have been shown to have few side effects and are remarkably well tolerated.

Unfortunately, cromolyn is not useful for acute attacks. In fact, it may take as long as two to three months to build up adequate therapeutic levels of it in the blood to be effective. These drugs are occasionally used alone, but more commonly their use is combined with

theophyllines or sympathomimetics. They have proven especially helpful when taken before workouts to control exercise-induced asthma.

Systemic corticosteroids, such as prednisone and prednisolone
(**Medrol**), especially when used for short periods of time under strict
medical supervision, are remarkably effective agents for reducing asthma symptoms. Among their many complex actions and interactions,
they are potent hormonelike antiinflammatory agents and stimulators
of CAMP. None of these agents should be confused with the much-
talked-about anabolic steroids used illegally by body-builders and
athletes to increase muscle mass and performance. Side effects of
prolonged, high-dose systemic corticosteroid therapy include the
development of cataracts, gastrointestinal ulcers, osteoporosis (loss of
bone calcium and vulnerability to fractures), potassium loss, and a
slightly increased susceptibility to infection. Owing to this potential
for adverse reactions, these medications are generally reserved for
more difficult or more severe cases of asthma.

Alternate-day steroid therapy has proven to be an important means
of maintenance control and of minimizing side effects in some chronic asthmatics. On an alternate-day steroid schedule, an individual
takes his dose every other day rather than every day. This regimen,
which has proven satisfactory in many patients requiring long-term
systemic corticosteroid therapy, permits a day's respite for restoration
of the body's normal hormonal balance, usually without significant
worsening of any symptoms on these days.

The use of corticosteroids locally, in spray form, is another way to
reduce potential side effects. **Azmacort**, **AeroBid**, **Beclovent**, and
Vanceril are four popular sprays containing different types of steroids.
Because they are inhaled directly into the breathing tubes rather than
ingested and carried in the bloodstream, steroid sprays essentially
work where they are most needed and have little effect on the rest of
the body. As a result, many physicians currently prefer them when
steroids are felt to be necessary.

Although antihistamines are the premier drugs for the treatment
of most allergies, they play only a small role in the management of
asthma. In fact, because of their ability to dry up secretions, antihis-

tamines were at one time avoided entirely for asthmatics because of the fear that they might worsen plugging and clogging of the small airways. More recent studies suggest otherwise, however. Nowadays, when an individual's seasonal or perennial allergies are believed to be a major trigger of asthma attacks, antihistamines may be prescribed as part of the treatment regimen for alleviating both the upper airway congestion and the nasal drip that can complicate an asthma attack.

Lastly, unless there is some concern about superimposed infection, antibiotics play a limited role in asthma therapy. In the event that you are feverish and are bringing up thick greenish or yellowish sputum, your doctor may prescribe a short course of any of a number of different antibiotics, including tetracyclines, erythromycins, and penicillin derivatives such as **Amoxicillin**. Bear in mind, however, that antibiotics are antibacterial agents and are of no benefit against viruses, the causes of the common cold, flu, and some cases of bronchitis. For this reason it is best to consult your doctor before taking any antibiotic that you may find in your medicine cabinet. You should make sure that you are using it appropriately and for the right kind of infection.

SOME USEFUL WARNING SIGNALS

Although in most cases asthma symptoms are relieved or well controlled by therapy, sometimes this is not the case. Because asthma can be a serious and even life-threatening disease, it is important for you to be able to recognize some of the warning signals of a severe attack.

Obtaining less than the expected degree of relief from your medications is probably one of the best tipoffs of an impending severe attack. Another is discovering that you are using your medications more and more frequently. Still another clue is observing a less-than-normal improvement in lung function as the day progresses. And finally, not improving at all or finding a worsening in lung function generally heralds a very severe attack. You should also regard seriously any increase in coughing, wheezing, and shortness of breath, and promptly seek medical attention.

Happily, only a tiny fraction of all asthmatics ever need emergency care. Thanks to the convenient and effective therapies currently available, most can expect to lead reasonably normal and productive lives.

CHAPTER SIX

WHEN YOUR MEAL PACKS A POWERFUL PUNCH: FOOD ALLERGIES

Although many people believe that foods are a major source of allergies, the fact is that the extent of the problem is still unknown. Some experts claim that true food allergies are relatively rare, while others contend that they are quite common. The statistics can be confusing. For example, some estimates place the incidence of food allergies in children somewhere between less than one-third of 1 percent to as high as 7.5 percent, while others put it at approximately 40 percent. And in adults, the numbers are no more definite; some experts estimate the incidence to be about 15 percent.

NONALLERGIC ADVERSE REACTIONS TO FOODS

Regardless of the precise figures, true allergies to foods—that is, those in which the immune system is involved—do indeed exist. The problem is that food allergies must be separated from a variety of other adverse reactions people can have to foods, those that are not immunologically related. These include food intolerances, druglike adverse reactions, and food poisoning. Because the signs and symptoms of any of these conditions can overlap with those of true allergic reactions to foods, diagnosing the cause of a suspected food-related problem can sometimes be difficult.

Food intolerances represent metabolic abnormalities related to the digestion of food rather than immunologic problems. Lactose intolerance is probably the best-known example of this type of reaction. Owing to a shortage of lactase, the intestinal enzyme that digests lactose found in milk and milk products, individuals with lactose intolerance suffer from abdominal cramping and diarrhea when they consume dairy products. African-Americans are especially prone to the condition, which is also prevalent in Mediterraneans and Asians. Symptoms result from the bacterial breakdown of the unmetabolized lactose in the bowel.

Druglike reactions to foods, or more correctly, *pharmacologic reactions*, occur whenever a particular substance in a food acts on the body like a drug. Caffeine, which is found in tea and coffee, is an excellent example of a food chemical that works in the body as a drug to keep you awake and more alert; when consumed in excessive quantities, it can make you "edgy." Nevertheless, the effect is purely chemical, not allergic in nature. Similarly, prunes, soybeans, and onions can trigger all kinds of gastrointestinal disturbances in some people on a purely chemical basis, as can the druglike chemicals in avocados, bananas, pineapple, and tomatoes. There are even substances in strawberries that are capable of nonallergically provoking hives and occasionally even life-threatening respiratory and blood pressure problems in susceptible people.

A toxic reaction, or *food poisoning*, is a third type of nonallergic adverse reaction to foods. Linked to the presence of germs in the food itself, this reaction may result from either the direct effects of the disease-producing germs themselves or from the specific druglike chemicals secreted by the germs. In either case, unlike a true allergic (immunologic) reaction that affects only susceptible individuals, a toxic reaction will affect all those who consume the affected food. *Salmonella* poisoning, which is the result of eating improperly cooked poultry, is a common example of the first type of toxic reaction. Victims typically suffer from nausea, vomiting, fever, and diarrhea.

Histamine poisoning, which is the result of consuming improperly refrigerated mackerel, swordfish, sardines, anchovies, and herring, is an example of the second type of reaction. Histamine is secreted by the bacteria that contaminate these foods, and rather than the germs themselves, the histamine is responsible for the flushing, hives, headache, and gastrointestinal problems that result.

TRUE FOOD ALLERGY

True food allergies involve the immune system and are of two types. By and large, they are of the immediate hypersensitivity variety (which was discussed in Chapter 1) that typically occurs within minutes of ingesting the culprit food and involves IgE antibodies, mast cells, basophils, and the release of histamine (as well as other mediators). The onset of these reactions may be so fast, in fact, that they may occur while the food is still in the mouth. Far less commonly, the food allergies are of the delayed hypersensitivity variety that involves T lymphocytes and takes many hours to develop.

Signs and Symptoms of Food Allergies

The signs and symptoms of a food allergy exhibited by a person depend on a number of factors, including the age of the individual, the quantity and quality of the food eaten, and the presence of other medical problems. Although the entire body may be affected, in general food allergies primarily target the gastrointestinal system, the skin, and, the least frequently, the respiratory system. Allergic symptoms therefore usually run the gamut from nausea, vomiting, and diarrhea to potentially fatal, multisystem shock. Why one organ system is the target site in one individual and not in another is still not known.

Not surprisingly, the gastrointestinal system, including the mouth and throat, is the primary target for food allergies. In fact, itching and swelling of the lips, oral mucous membranes, palate, and throat can occasionally occur as soon as the food passes through. Fortunately, such reactions are usually temporary and are not always followed by additional allergic manifestations. However, after being digested in the stomach and intestines, some offending foods will go on to provoke other GI complaints such as abdominal distention, cramps, gassiness, diarrhea, nausea, and vomiting.

The skin is the next most common target organ for food allergies. Typical adverse reactions include acute, and less often chronic, itchy hive reactions or severe giant hive reactions, known as *angioedema*. It is important to note that flare-ups of asthma, eczema, or rhinitis conditions may also occur in response to food allergy, especially in children; this connection is much less certain in adults.

Some of the Common Troublemakers

While food allergies are more common in children, they may develop at any age. In general, however, they tend to diminish in severity or disappear entirely later in life. Hereditary factors have been implicated in their development, and individuals with a personal or family history of atopy (asthma, hay fever, or eczema) appear at somewhat greater risk for them. Although any food is potentially allergenic, the foods most commonly implicated in immediate hypersensitivity reactions include eggs, milk, wheat, peanuts, soybeans, chicken, fish, nuts, shellfish, and mollusks.

The complexity of our modern diets makes the avoidance of food allergens more difficult than you might think. Without your knowing it, you may be eating all kinds of derivatives of foods that you are allergic to. For example, if you have an allergy to corn, you must also be wary of corn-derived additives such as caramel coloring, citric acid, xanthin gum, lecithin, modified food starch, and malto-dextrin. And if you are super-sensitive to corn, you may run into problems from just licking a postage stamp whose sticky side is coated with a corn derivative.

Milk is another good example. Besides being in numerous dairy products such as creams, cheeses, and yogurts, it may also be found, though less obviously, in caramel coloring, lactic acid, and calcium lactate. Soy, too, which is found in texturized vegetable protein as well as the soybean by-products of glycerin and tocopherols, may be difficult to avoid. What is clear is that just knowing the specific foods you are allergic to and avoiding them may not be enough. You must also know their derivatives and in which products they may be found.

Interestingly, despite the widely held notion that tomatoes and citrus fruits are frequent food allergens, well-designed medical studies have not supported this contention to date. Moreover, some people most certainly develop hives after eating strawberries, but no studies have been able to demonstrate an allergic (IgE antibody) basis for the reaction.

FOOD CONTAMINANTS

Allergies to contaminants in certain foods must be distinguished from true allergies to the foods themselves. For example, an allergic reaction to cheeses, dried fruits, yogurt, or wine may not actually represent an allergy to these foods per se but to the presence of certain molds that often contaminate them. Unsavory as it may sound, insect parts, which occasionally find their way into certain spices and other foods, can provoke allergies and lead to the mistaken assumption that the particular food item is at fault. And, finally, it may not be the milk itself that is responsible for all cases of supposed "milk allergy" but the bacitracin, tetracycline, or penicillin that finds its way into our milk supply after it has been fed to the herds to prevent cattle diseases.

FOOD ADDITIVES

Despite what has been said, it might appear that isolating the cause of a potential food allergy is a fairly easy task. You might be tempted to reason: "I ate applesauce. I broke out in hives. I am therefore allergic to apples." Unfortunately, this may not be true. These days, foods contain additives of all kinds, and this can make determining the specific allergenic agent a very difficult piece of detective work. Unlike contaminants, additives, as the term suggests, are chemicals that have been added intentionally to a product for one reason or another.

In the broadest terms, a food additive is any substance that becomes part of a food product by being added directly or indirectly. For example, many foods are fortified with vitamins and minerals to maintain or improve their nutritional value. Others contain additives to prevent spoilage and to maintain freshness, color, and flavor. Still others are used to make foods more appealing to the eye and to the palate. Finally, a wide variety of chemicals are added to foods to give body or texture, or to enhance preparability.

According to the Public Health Service, approximately twenty-eight hundred substances are intentionally added to foods to produce a desired effect. Moreover, as many as ten thousand other ingredients or ingredient mixtures may be added to foods during processing, packaging, or storage. The most common food additives are sugar, salt and corn syrup, citric acid, baking soda, vegetable colors, mustard, and pepper. Taken together, these substances currently account by weight for greater than 98 percent of all the food additives used in the United States.

The following is a brief description of some common additive ingredients and the more frequent kinds of adverse reactions that have been associated with them:

1. Aspartame (**NutraSweet**), a non-nutritive sweetener found in numerous foods and beverages, has been linked with ordinary hives as well as a severe form of hives known as *angioedema*. In 1985 I reported the first proven case in the world's literature of the development of numerous nodules in the legs of a young woman who had consumed large amounts of aspartame-containing soda. The condition was fortunately reversible and

entirely cleared once the patient stopped consuming the aspartame beverages.

2. *Butylated hydroxyanisole* (BHA) and *Butylated hydroxytoluene-butylated hydroxyanisole* (BHT-BHA), common antioxidants used in cereals and other grain products, have been linked to hives and other skin rashes.

3. *FD&C Yellow #5* (*tartrazine*), a food coloring found in many foods and beverages, is another known hive provoker.

4. *Monosodium glutamate* (MSG), a popular flavor enhancer, especially for Chinese foods and also found in many fresh and packaged products, frozen dinners, and gourmet seasonings, has been associated with a variety of adverse reactions, including aggravation of asthma, burning sensations in the back of the neck, chest tightness, diarrhea, facial pain, headache, and nausea.

5. *Nitrates* and *Nitrites*, which serve as preservatives, flavor enhancers, and colorants in processed foods such as bacon, bologna, frankfurters, salami, sausages, and smoked fish, are known to trigger headaches and hives.

6. The *parabens*, including *butyl-, ethyl-, methyl-,* and *propyl-,* and their relative, *sodium benzoate*, are common preservatives used in many foods and drugs. They are well-recognized causes of itching, pain, skin rashes, and swelling.

7. The *sulfites*, including *bisulfite, metabisulfite, potassium sulfite, sodium sulfite,* and *sulfur dioxide*, are another large group of chemicals used as preservatives and container sanitizers. They are found in canned, frozen, and dehydrated fruits; beer, wine, wine coolers, and cider; pizza, processed grains, and packaged potato products; prescription drugs; salad dressings; soups; vegetables; shrimp; tea mixes, and Mexican food. They have been linked to such diverse reactions as abdominal cramps, asthma, chest tightness, diarrhea, elevated pulse rate, hives, light-headedness, lowered blood pressure, and vomiting.

DIAGNOSING FOOD ALLERGIES

If you find, for example, that every time you drink milk or eat peanuts, you break out with hives, you might strongly suspect an allergy to these foods. And if you have a personal or family history of atopic eczema, hay fever, asthma, or hive reactions to nonfood allergens, then the possibility of food allergies is more likely. On the other hand, because the signs and symptoms of certain skin, gastrointestinal, and respiratory diseases may mimic those of food allergies, such conditions must be excluded by means of a careful medical history and physical examination *before* a food allergy is diagnosed.

After a preliminary evaluation has been made and it has been determined that foods may be the culprits, a number of diagnostic tests are available to help cinch the diagnosis. Scratch tests involve making a series of small scratches on the skin and placing minute amounts of test food allergens on them to see whether an allergy is provoked. Redness and swelling at the test site indicate allergy. In general, tests for eggs, nuts, fish, milk, peanuts, and wheat correlate fairly well with allergic symptoms.

Unfortunately, this is not the case with many other foods. In other words, a skin test may indicate that you are allergic to a specific food. But if you experience no symptoms when you eat that food, you are *not* allergic to it. Doctors refer to this as a *false positive result*, and as many as 30 percent of normal individuals may have false positive skin test reactions to various foods. On the other hand, a negative skin test result—that is, one where a food allergen does not provoke a reaction—is a far more reliable finding for excluding a particular food as a possible allergic culprit.

Intradermal testing is another form of skin testing; however, it is seldom used nowadays in food testing. In this type of skin test, the suspected material is injected directly into the skin, and the test sites are observed for redness and swelling. The test is no more useful than conventional scratch testing, but because of a real risk of provoking a severe, life-threatening allergic reaction, it is no longer recommended.

Although less sensitive than skin testing for discovering allergies, RAST, a relatively expensive blood test, may be used to determine the presence of IgE antibodies to specific food allergens. The major advantage of this test is its safety, which is a clear benefit when individuals who have experienced potentially life-threatening reactions to foods are being tested.

Food challenges, in which the offending substances are given to the patient under strict medical supervision (usually in a hospital), are the only truly definitive tests for food allergies. Challenges are performed in one of three ways: open challenges, single-blind challenges, and double-blind challenges. In open challenges, both the patient and the physician are aware which allergen is being given. Because this test is more subjective, it is the least exacting of the three methods. In a single-blind test, only the patient knows what he or she is getting, making the test somewhat more objective. In a double-blind test, the most objective of the three, suspected food allergens and placebos are placed in gelatin capsules, and neither the patient nor the doctor knows which is being given. Allergy symptoms provoked in the double-blind setting can be taken as firm evidence of a true adverse reaction to a food. None of these tests needs to be performed if there is a clear-cut history of allergic symptoms that can be related to a specific food or foods. In other words, if you are certain that your respiratory symptoms or the swelling of your lips, tongue, or face began shortly after eating a certain food, you would generally not need these tests.

Elimination diets have also been used for many years in the diagnosis of food allergies. As the term suggests, these tests consist of eliminating potential food troublemakers from the diet entirely and then reintroducing them one at a time to see if they cause symptoms. Elimination diets usually exclude the following foods from the diet: cinnamon, chocolate (including colas), citrus fruits (grapefruit, lemons, and oranges), corn (including cereals, flour, meal, oil, starch, and syrup), eggs, food coloring and preservatives, grains (barley, millet, oats, rice, and wheat), legumes (beans, peas, peanuts, and soybeans), and tomatoes. More restrictive elimination diets permit only applesauce, bananas, lamb, and rice to be eaten.

If symptoms persist on a strict elimination diet, it is unlikely that the restricted foods are the problem. But if they disappear when a particular food is eliminated and then return when it is reintroduced into the diet, the cause-and-effect link is strengthened. Although this form of testing is frequently tedious and time-consuming, it has the advantage of greater safety when compared to some of the other methods already described.

Two tests deserve special mention because they have proven to be entirely useless and nothing more than a waste of time and money. The first is called *cytotoxic leukocyte testing*. According to the theory behind this test, food allergens possess the ability to lower your natural white blood cell (*leukocyte*) count or to induce derangements in their functioning. Proponents of the test believe that such abnormalities can be determined by either giving an individual the suspected food allergen and then drawing a blood sample to look for the changes, or adding the food allergen directly to a test tube sample of the patient's blood to look for the effects.

Sublingual testing is likewise of no proven value. In this test, droplets of increasing concentrations of food extracts are placed under the tongue (sublingually) until a dosage that provokes allergic symptoms is finally reached. Once this information is obtained, various concentrations of the food allergens are then continually administered sublingually, usually several times a week, in hopes of "neutralizing" the allergy. Neither cytotoxic leucocyte testing nor sublingual testing has demonstrated usefulness for either diagnosis or therapy, and both have been abandoned by most reputable physicians.

PREVENTION AND TREATMENT

There is some evidence that reducing the exposure of infants to food allergens may prevent the later development of certain allergic disorders. In one recent study reported in the respected medical journal *Lancet*, a group of nursing mothers was instructed to avoid eggs, fish, milk, nuts, and other potential allergens from their own diet as well as from that of their baby's until the child was between nine and twelve months. Researchers found a significantly reduced incidence of asthma, eczema, and food intolerance in this group as compared to a control group of mothers and infants who maintained a normal diet. While the study suggested that such dietary changes might reduce the short-term risk of allergic disorders in infants, the study group was small, and no conclusions could be drawn about the possible long-term benefits. (If you are nursing a baby, you should consult your child's pediatrician before making any changes in your diet or that of your baby's.)

As harsh as it may seem, the only specific "treatment" for food allergies, once you have developed them, is prevention by strict avoidance. But you must do more than merely avoid eating the food to which you are allergic; you must also watch out for foods that are relatives of the culprit. For example, if you are allergic to cashews, you may also be allergic to mangoes and pistachio nuts and should be cautious with these foods as well. Or if you are allergic to crabs, you should be cautious when consuming crayfish, lobster, or shrimp. Doctors call the problem *cross-reactivity*. You might want to ask your doctor for a list of related food allergens, and, in addition, you might benefit from the advice of a skilled dietician regarding menu planning.

Happily, having to eliminate certain foods from your diet because of allergies does not necessarily mean that you will be never be able to eat them again. Some problem foods that evoke symptoms when consumed in large quantities may cause no significant problems when eaten in tiny amounts or as an ingredient in the preparation of other dishes. And there are some food allergens that cannot be eaten raw without causing symptoms but that do not induce symptoms when eaten thoroughly cooked. Also, best of all, some people, particularly children, entirely outgrow their allergies in time.

When an allergy attack is already under way, however, antihistamines, such as those used to treat hay fever and perennial allergies, may also be used for controlling food allergy symptoms. More severe reactions that are unresponsive to antihistamines may require the additional prescription of an antiinflammatory steroid, such as prednisone. At present the use of oral cromolyn sodium for food allergies to stabilize mast cells and prevent histamine release remains controversial and has not been approved by the FDA.

If in the past you have experienced a potentially life-threatening reaction to a food, you would do well to be alert to the danger signs of serious food allergies. If you experience, during or shortly after eating, the rapid onset of breathing difficulties or a feeling that your throat is closing, you should seek *immediate* medical attention. You should also carry with you a small emergency kit for the self-injection of epinephrine (**Adrenalin**). Epinephrine-containing kits, such as **EpiPen** or **Ana-Kit**, are sold in most pharmacies and are the same as those carried by people with life-threatening reactions to bee or wasp stings. Unfortunately, in contrast to their generally good track record in dealing with hay fever allergies, allergy shots have not proven helpful in the vast majority of food allergy cases.

THE CANDIDA CONNECTION

No chapter on food allergies would be complete without some mention of the organism *Candida*. *Candida albicans* (or monilia, as it is also known) is a common yeast organism that inhabits the mouth, gastrointestinal system, and vagina. Under ordinary circumstances these organisms cause no problems, but after a course of antibiotics or oral steroids, they tend to proliferate and cause the burning, redness, and discharge of yeast vaginitis, a condition that in most cases is easily treated successfully with antifungal agents.

In the early 1980s, the notion became popular that an excessive growth of native *Candida* or an abnormally increased sensitivity to its presence in the abdomen was responsible for a wide variety of vague, nonspecific complaints and symptoms. These included a general feeling of illness, anxiety, depression, excessive tiredness, headaches, heightened premenstrual tension, irritability, and trouble concentrating. The theory initially met with appeal, especially in lay, nutrition, and holistic circles, but most of the evidence supporting it was founded on the testimonials of individuals. To date, hard scientific evidence has failed to substantiate the *Candida* connection. For one thing, the skin tests and stool cultures for *Candida* routinely used for diagnosing the presence of the organism are positive in more than 90 percent of people because the organism is found normally in just about everyone.

Even when it comes to treatment, the results were disappointing when nystatin, an anti-*Candida* drug, was given, in controlled medical studies, to patients who supposedly had *Candida* sensitivity. Researchers found that patients treated with the drug fared no better than those treated with placebo (sugar) pills. And finally, the use of yeast elimination diets, often strongly recommended by adherents of the *Candida* connection, likewise have proved of little overall value. Fortunately, both the testing for *Candida* and the prescription of nystatin and *Candida* elimination diets are not particularly harmful in themselves.

Few physicians continue to give much credence to the *Candida* theory and instead look for other allergic or nonallergic causes for their patients' complaints. If you decide to explore this avenue for relief of your symptoms, however, you should keep in mind that you may be not only wasting your time and money but delaying your receipt of a proper diagnosis and treatment for your problems.

CHAPTER SEVEN

WARNING: THE MEDICATION YOU TAKE MAY BE DANGEROUS TO YOUR HEALTH

J ust because your doctor has given you a prescription drug for your cough or your pharmacist has recommended some one-hundred-year-old all-time favorite OTC remedy for your upset stomach does not mean you won't have a bad reaction to the medication. Unfortunately, in our less than perfect world there is just no such thing as a medication (prescription or otherwise) that cannot cause adverse reactions in some people. While the exact number of untoward reactions that occur is not known, it is estimated that the drug-related complication rate in hospitalized patients alone is between 6 percent and 15 percent. No doubt a far greater number occur at home and thus go unreported.

NONALLERGIC DRUG REACTIONS

Not all adverse reactions to medications are allergic (immune-system linked) in nature. In fact, true allergies to medications probably comprise less than one-quarter of all hospital-based adverse drug reactions. The majority of unwanted effects are brought about by several non-immunologic means, including the following:

1. Direct toxic reactions
2. Impairment of the body's germ-fighting capability
3. Suppression of the body's normal protective germ population
4. Undesirable interactions between medications taken for different conditions
5. Idiosyncratic reactions

You may be wondering what practical difference it makes whether or not an adverse drug reaction (ADR) is allergic in origin. Such information is of more than just passing interest and can sometimes even be critical to a patient's life. To appreciate this, imagine that you have developed an allergy to a particular drug, and your doctor has informed you that you must never take that drug again. Now imagine that sometime afterward you fall ill with a condition that would normally necessitate treatment with that drug. If you are lucky, the condition will be one for which many different kinds of drugs have been found useful; in this instance your particular drug allergy may not be very important. On the other hand, if your condition is one for which the drug you are allergic to is the only one used for treatment or is the best one for the job, the fact that you are allergic to it may be critically important. Not uncommonly, this is the case with people who are allergic to penicillin, insulin, or the iodine-containing contrast material used in many X-ray diagnostic procedures, where no satisfactory substitutes are available.

Direct toxic reactions to medications generally result from intentional or inadvertent overdosage. Even a brief listing of the more common direct toxic reactions would fill a book much larger than this. The *Physician's Desk Reference*, found in many libraries and used by many physicians, is a valuable source of this kind of information. One example of a reaction is ringing in the ears; this is related to salicylism and is a common side effect of taking too much aspirin. Another reaction is vertigo, the sense of the room spinning around; this may result from an excessive dose of the antibiotic minocycline. Nausea and heart rhythm abnormalities may result from an overdose of theophylline.

Occasionally, toxic doses of a drug occur from an abnormal buildup within the body rather than from taking too much of it at one time. Since most medications are either broken down in the liver before excretion from the body or are eliminated directly through the kidneys into the urine, any coexisting damage or disease to these two organs can lead to drug overaccumulation and toxicity. For example, when the kidneys are not functioning optimally, the dose of certain diuretics (such as **Lasix**) must be reduced in order to prevent toxic damage to the auditory system, a situation that can lead to permanent hearing loss. Similarly astemizole (**Hismanal**), a popular nonsedating antihistamine that is metabolized by the liver, must be administered in much lower doses or avoided entirely in people with liver problems; otherwise, it can provoke serious heart rhythm abnormalities.

Alterations in the body's ability to fight infection—or, as doctor's call it, *immune system impairment*—is another potential nonallergic side effect of certain drugs. For example, many anticancer (antineoplastic) drugs as well as systemic corticosteroids (such as prednisone), besides their beneficial effects, unfortunately also suppress the body's natural ability to fight off infections. This leaves the patient vulnerable to a wide variety of viral, fungal, and bacterial germs. This weakened ability to fight off infection during treatment is often the direct cause of death. In addition, both kinds of drugs interfere with the body's structural repair and blood-clotting mechanisms, promoting the development of widespread black-and-blue skin rashes called *purpura*.

The inadvertent upset of the body's delicate equilibrium between "good" germs (those that harmlessly colonize various regions of the body) and potential troublemakers (those just waiting to cause infection) is another important drug side effect. Whether we like to believe it or not, our body cavities are ordinarily teeming with all kinds of germs that coexist in a delicate equilibrium with one another. Most benefit us by outcompeting the more harmful organisms while their own numbers remain too small to cause us any significant harm. The familiar *lactobacilli* that normally colonize the vagina are good examples of this type of helpful organism. Normal numbers of these bacteria prevent the overgrowth of *Candida*.

Problems arise when, for example, you need an antibiotic for either a gum or a urinary tract infection. At the same time the drug kills the undesirable germs in your mouth or urine, it also suppresses the populations of the "good" germs in other areas of the body, allowing "bad" ones to achieve a foothold and cause problems. The onset of yeast vaginitis in women taking penicillin, tetracycline, or erythromycin is a classic example of this scenario, which is why so many women dread taking any of these drugs. Clindamycin-associated *pseudomembranous colitis* is a more serious example of this kind of adverse drug reaction. By suppressing normal gut organisms, clindamycin permits the overgrowth of the toxin-producing bacteria responsible for this potentially life-threatening colon inflammation and diarrheal disease.

An idiosyncratic reaction, yet another form of nonimmunologic ADR, refers to any adverse reaction whose underlying mechanism for occurrence is unknown. Fortunately idiosyncratic drug reactions are relatively rare, but they may be provoked by even tiny amounts of a culprit medication (that is, amounts well below the therapeutic dose). Examples include the anemia caused by phenytoin (**Dilantin**), the widely prescribed anticonvulsant; the nerve cell inflammation seen with isoniazid (**INH**), currently the number one antibiotic against tuberculosis; and the bone marrow suppressive effects on red blood cell production of the broad-spectrum antibiotic chloramphenicol (**Chloromycetin**).

Finally, another source of nonallergic problems are undesirable medication interactions. For example, astemizole (**Hismanal**) and terfenadine (**Seldane**) should not be given to individuals who are taking erythromycin or ketoconazole (**Nizoral**). There is a significantly increased risk of provoking serious heartbeat irregularities when these agents are combined. They should also be used cautiously by anyone taking diuretics because they, too, by altering salt concentrations in the blood, also occasionally pose a risk of precipitating heart rhythm abnormalities.

These are just a few examples of the thousands of potential adverse drug interactions that a doctor must keep in mind when prescribing medications for persons with multiple medical conditions. Obviously it is extremely important to tell your doctor about any OTC or prescription medications you are taking, including headache pills and vitamins.

TRUE DRUG ALLERGIES

By definition, an allergic reaction to a medication is caused by some kind of interaction between the immune system and the drug. In general, the molecules of many drugs by themselves are too small to engender an allergic reaction. When combined with proteins in the tissues or bloodstream, however, the molecules of these drugs or their metabolic breakdown products become large enough to provoke an allergy.

Evidence suggests that in some cases there may be a family predisposition for the development of drug allergies. For example, there is ordinarily a chance of about one in five thousand of experiencing a severe reaction to sulfonamides or anticonvulsants. But if another family member has had a reaction to one of these drugs, the risk jumps to one in four. For this reason it is especially important to inform physicians about any family history of drug allergies.

As a rule, a true drug allergy does not begin with the first exposure to a new drug. It usually takes between seven and twenty-one days for the drug-protein complexes in the body to provoke the hypersensitivity. The interval between the first exposure to a particular drug and the onset of allergy symptoms is known as the period of *sensitization*. During this critical period the drug-protein complexes interact with the immune system to stimulate antibodies and a variety of immune system cells (see Chapter 1). Unfortunately, the frequency of drug allergies increases with age, so we can all expect to develop an allergy to two or three different drugs as we grow older.

The phenomenon of *cross-reactivity* is another important aspect of drug allergies. What this means is that by developing an allergy to one medication, you may become automatically allergic to others to which that one is chemically related. For example, we know that a great deal of cross-reactivity exists between the various anticonvulsant drugs that are currently available. In fact, about 75 percent of individuals allergic to one member of this group will have a reaction to all of them, and the other 25 percent will have a reaction to at least one other member of the group. In a similar way, persons allergic to penicillin or to one of its derivatives are very likely to be allergic to all penicillin derivatives.

Once you have become sensitized (that is, you have developed an allergy), you usually have the allergy symptoms each time you take the drug. And, frequently, each successive episode is worse than the previous one. In severe cases allergy symptoms occur within hours of the first dose.

Types of Drug-induced Immune Reactions

Based on differing underlying mechanisms, doctors usually divide drug allergies into four main types: immediate hypersensitivity allergies, immune complex disease, cytotoxic responses, and delayed hypersensitivity reactions.

Generally occurring anywhere from instantly to within the first six hours after exposure to the culprit medication, immediate hypersensitivity drug reactions involve IgE antibodies, mast cells, and the release of large amounts of chemical mediators (see Chapter 1) that are responsible for the symptoms. These reactions may be severe and even life-threatening. Penicillin, when administered either intramuscularly or intravenously, is perhaps the best known cause of this type of severe reaction, but by no means the sole cause. Many other types of antibiotics, adrenocorticotropic hormone (ACTH), insulin, flu vaccine, tetanus toxoid, and gamma globulin may also provoke immediate hypersensitivity drug reactions and profound shock.

Immune-complex disease, once called serum sickness disease, is a second kind of drug-induced allergy. In this type of reaction, small-sized drug-antibody molecular complexes float in the bloodstream until they are deposited in the tiny blood vessels of many important organs. Once there, they attract other blood proteins and initiate a cascade of events, culminating in significant inflammation and damage to the surrounding tissues and organs. Symptoms include fever, rash, hives, tender black-and-blue nodules in the skin, swollen glands, and joint pains. Drugs commonly linked to this type of allergy include penicillin, sulfa drugs, phenytoin (**Dilantin**), aspirin, streptomycin, hydralazine (**Apresoline**), procainamide (**Pronestyl**), isoniazid (**INH**), propylthiouracil, and chlorpromazine (**Thorazine**).

Cytotoxic reactions (which literally mean those that are poisonous to cells) are a third kind of drug allergy. In simplest terms, the offending drug alone or the drug bound to an antibody attaches to the surface of specific target cells—for example, red blood cells—and initiates their destruction. Drugs that may precipitate anemia (a low blood count) in this manner include penicillin, quinidine (**Quinaglute**), quinine, aspirin, and cephalosporin antibiotics (**Keflex, Velosef,** and **Duricef**). Destruction of platelets, the cells needed for normal blood coagulation, has been reported with quinine, quinidine, acetaminophen (**Tylenol**), and sulfa drugs. And lastly, white blood cell destruction has been linked to phenylbutazone (**Butazolidin**), phenothiazines (for example, **Thorazine**), sulfa drugs, phenytoin (**Dilantin**), and tolbutamide (**Orinase**), among others.

Finally, drugs may cause allergy by a fourth immunologic mechanism known as delayed hypersensitivity, which involves the participation of sensitized lymphocytes. Within the skin, delayed reactions manifest themselves as allergic contact dermatitis (see Chapter 8). Neomycin, bacitracin, parabens, propylene glycol, and PABA are examples of common ingredients found in many OTC and prescription items that are known to cause contact allergies. Although it occurs less often, a delayed hypersensitivity reaction may also involve other organs. For example, nitrofurantoin (**Furadantin**), penicillin, and phenytoin (**Dilantin**) have been known to cause delayed hypersensitivity inflammation in the lungs.

SIGNS AND SYMPTOMS

The specific set of allergy symptoms caused by a medication depends on the organs affected. In some cases symptoms start soon after therapy begins; in other cases the symptoms begin when the person is well into therapy; in still others the symptoms begin after therapy has been discontinued. Occasionally they disappear spontaneously even though the drug is continued; but most often, the drug must be stopped for the condition to clear.

Skin Eruptions

Most drug allergies involve the skin in some way, and many drugs are capable of eliciting more than one type of skin reaction. Itching, small hives, massive hives, red blotches, measlelike rashes, and eczema conditions are all well-recognized complications of certain topical or systemic drugs. Less common drug-related skin problems include fixed drug eruptions (where a patch or several patches of redness and discoloration appear in the same exact location each time a particular drug is ingested); purpura (black-and-blue marks of varying sizes); blistering eruptions; phototoxic reactions (heightened sensitivity to ultraviolet light leading to severe sunburns); photoallergic reactions (ultraviolet light combines with the drug to provoke a true allergic eczema); erythema multiforme (an exaggerated form of hives), erythema nodosum (deep, painful nodules, typically over the lower extremities), and exfoliative dermatitis (a red, scaly rash that covers more than 90 percent of the skin surface, including the scalp).

With good reason, *toxic epidermal necrolysis*, a frequently fatal condition in which large sheets of skin and mucous membrane tissue literally slough away, is the most feared skin manifestation of drug allergy. Skin allergies of various kinds have been tied to penicillin and its derivatives (such as ampicillin, amoxicillin, and dicloxacillin), trimethoprim-sulfa antibiotics (**Septra** and **Bactrim**), sulfisoxazole (**Gantrisin** and **Gantanol**), cephalosporins (**Keflex, Velosef,** and

Duricef), barbiturates (such as phenobarbital), and quinidine (Quinaglute), among numerous others.

Drug Fever

Fever can be the sole manifestation of a drug allergy or may accompany skin eruptions and other organ symptoms. It is believed to be related to the release of *pyrogens* (temperature-raising chemical mediators) from certain kinds of white blood cells. When fever is the only symptom, it usually begins sometime between the seventh and tenth day following the start of drug treatment. Characteristically, discontinuing the drug leads to a return to normal temperature, but reintroducing the drug quickly leads to the return of the fever. Penicillin is a common fever producer, as are quinidine (**Quinaglute**), procainamide (**Pronestyl**), barbiturates (such as **Seconal**), and phenytoin (**Dilantin**).

Respiratory Tract Reactions

Like the skin, the respiratory system can react adversely to drugs in a number of ways: fluid buildup in the lungs, infiltration by lymphocytes and other kinds of white cells, inflammation and swelling of the air sacs or of the walls separating them, formation of scar tissue, and the development of acute, potentially life-threatening airway obstruction. Methotrexate (an antiarthritis, anticancer, and antipsoriasis agent), nitrofurantoin (such as **Furadantin**, an antibiotic for bladder infection), sulfasalazine (such as **Azulfidine**, an anticolitis drug), and cromolyn sodium (**Intal**) are all known causes of a drug-induced pneumonialike lung allergy. Hydrochlorothiazide (such as **HydroDIURIL**, a water pill), heroin, and methadone may all cause *pulmonary edema* (fluid in the lungs), and aspirin may cause life-threatening bronchospasm in susceptible individuals (as discussed below).

Liver Reactions

Certain drugs have been linked to adverse liver reactions. Most often the symptoms are due either to bile duct congestion and backup within the liver or to direct injury to the liver cells themselves—that is, a chemical hepatitis. Certain anticonvulsive (antiepilepsy) medications, erythromycin estolate (**Ilosone**), gold salts (**Myochrisine**), halothane (a general anesthetic agent), indomethacin (**Indocin**), isoniazid (**INH**), ketoconazole (**Nizoral**), methyldopa (**Aldomet**), phenothiazines (such as **Thorazine** and **Mellaril**), sulfa drugs (such as **Gantrisin**), and certain thyroid medications (propylthiouracil, for example) have all been associated with liver abnormalities. Although postulated, allergic mechanisms have not been conclusively demonstrated in any of these instances. In most cases, fortunately, the abnormalities completely subside when the offending drug is withdrawn.

Kidney Problems

Considering that the kidney is the body's main waste filter, it is hardly surprising that it is occasionally adversely affected by the drugs we take. The delicate filtering portions of the kidney and the tissues immediately surrounding them are particularly susceptible to dam-age. Gold injections, methicillin, large doses of penicillin G, cephalosporins, nonsteroidal inflammatory agents (such as **Anaprox**, **Motrin**, and **Nuprin**), and phenytoin (**Dilantin**) have all been linked to kidney reactions.

Swollen Lymph Nodes

Generalized lymph node enlargement, or as doctors call it, *lymphadenopathy*, has been reported in individuals receiving long-term phenytoin (**Dilantin**), sulfonamide, and penicillin therapy. Believed allergic in nature, lymph gland enlargement can occasionally be so pronounced as to be initially confused with a malignancy. In most instances, discontinuing the culprit medication leads to complete resolution of the problem.

Blood Problems

Drugs can damage the blood system in a variety of ways. As part of cytotoxic reactions, they may induce anemia by destroying red corpuscles. Or they may lead to bruising problems by interfering with platelets, one of the blood's most important clotting components. In a serum sicknesslike fashion, they may inflame and damage the blood vessels themselves in the skin, joints, and kidneys, resulting in a condition technically known as *allergic vasculitis*. Allopurinol (an antigout medication such as **Zyloprim**), hydantoin (**Dilantin**), penicillin, and sulfa have all been associated with this type of kidney reaction.

Anaphylaxis

Fortunately a relatively rare adverse drug reaction, anaphylaxis is the most dreaded of all allergies to medications. Symptoms usually begin within about half an hour of taking the culprit medication. At first the victim usually complains of feeling anxious and tense. This is often succeeded by the onset of a vicious, splitting headache, which in turn is quickly followed by tissue swelling and airway blockage within the respiratory system, fluid accumulation in the lungs, a lowering of blood pressure, heart rhythm abnormalities, and finally heart stoppage. If emergency measures are not instituted immediately, death usually results. Penicillin and anesthetics (local and general) are examples of medications that may provoke anaphylaxis in susceptible individuals.

DRUGS DESERVING SPECIAL NOTE

Because of their widespread use as well as their well-known propensities for triggering allergic reactions, aspirin, penicillin, and local anesthetics deserve special mention.

Aspirin

Aspirin and other salicylates are well-known causes of upset stomach, ulcers, easy bruisability, and liver irritations, but they are also associated with a number of immediate problems that appear to be similar to hypersensitivity, including hives, giant hive reactions, and anaphylaxis. In addition, approximately 15 percent of aspirin-sensitive asthmatics are also sensitive to the food and drug coloring agent tartrazine (FD&C #5), which is used to give the yellow-orange color to many drinks, cereals, and medications.

But probably the best-recognized aspirin-related syndrome involves the gradual development of rhinitis and sinusitis, followed by the growth of nasal polyps and the development of severe, difficult-to-control asthma, the so-called rhinitis-sinusitis-polyposis-asthma syndrome. This constellation of problems typically develops in otherwise healthy, middle-aged individuals who have never had trouble with aspirin before. Once the condition develops, however, it generally persists even when aspirin is discontinued. Those with the syndrome must avoid not only aspirin but other nonsteroidal antiinflammatory agents, such as indomethacin, ibuprofen, naproxen, phenylbutazone (such as **Indocin**, **Motrin**, **Naprosyn**, and **Butazolidin**, respectively). However, both sodium aminosalicylate (**Tubasal**) and choline magnesium salicylate (**Trilisate**), despite their chemical similarity to aspirin, as well as acetaminophen (**Tylenol**) may be substituted for aspirin and other nonsteroidal antiinflammatory agents whenever a medication is needed for pain and or to reduce fever. Obviously, for the reasons given, if you know that you are aspirin-sensitive, you would do well to read all food product labels carefully and to check with your physician or pharmacist before taking any new medication.

Penicillin

From what has already been said, you should not be surprised to learn that penicillin is a leading provoker of adverse drug reactions. In fact, about 2 percent of people are estimated to be allergic to penicillin, and more than six hundred people die each year from penicillin allergy in the United States and Canada alone. While less threatening conditions—small hives, giant hives, and other itchy skin rashes—make up the bulk of penicillin reactions, death occurs in about one in every one hundred thousand times the drug is administered. As a rule the drug appears to be about twice as likely to provoke allergic reactions when given intramuscularly or intravenously rather than when taken orally.

Unfortunately, the story does not end there. If you are allergic to penicillin, you are also very likely to be allergic to its derivatives. These include amoxicillin, ampicillin, dicloxacillin, and methicillin, all of which are commonly used antibiotics. Furthermore, since there is a known cross-reactivity between the penicillins and another, very popular group of broad-spectrum antibiotics, the cephalosporins (such as **Keflex, Ceclor, Velosef,** and **Duricef**), these agents should also be avoided by penicillin-allergic persons or used with special caution.

If you've had an allergic reaction to penicillin in the past, you may take some comfort in knowing that approximately 50 percent of penicillin-allergic people lose their allergy after five years and about 80 percent lose it after ten years. This makes it possible for them once again to take the drug (or its derivatives) if needed. Skin testing is an excellent method for detecting IgE- anti-penicillin antibodies and therefore for determining whether a person who had an adverse reaction earlier is still allergic or has "outgrown" the allergy.

Testing is usually reserved for persons suffering from an infection for which penicillin is the drug of choice and for which there exists no comparably effective substitute. Two penicillin derivatives, peni-cilloyl polylysine (PPL, Pre-pen) and penicillin G (PG), are generally used. Patients are first given a prick test, and if there is no adverse reaction, they are then tested intradermally—that is, small amounts of the test materials are introduced under the skin to see if local skin reactions result. Virtually all persons at risk for allergic reactions to penicillin are skin-test positive: They react with redness, itching, and hiving at the test sites.

Desensitization methods (procedures for overcoming penicillin allergy) have been developed for treating allergy-proven individuals who must receive penicillin. Under strict observation, such patients are given (usually orally) increasing doses of penicillin every five to fifteen minutes, starting with very small amounts. The protocol is con-tinued until full therapeutic doses can be tolerated without provoking any allergy symptoms. Unfortunately, desensitization is not uniform-ly successful.

On a related note, oral desensitization to trimethroprim/sulfa (**Septra** and **Bactrim**), another important and widely used antibiotic, was achieved in a small study group of sixty-two HIV-positive patients who had previously developed drug rashes or fever while receiving the drug. These results are of no small importance considering that aller-gies to the drug occur in about half of all HIV-infected persons and that the medication has been shown to be highly effective for pre-venting a relatively common, potentially life-threatening form of pneumonia in these individuals. The desensitization protocol involves giving increasing doses of the antibiotic every six hours for eight days until therapeutic levels are achieved without any untoward reaction.

Local Anesthetics

Because they are used so often in dental and ambulatory surgery, local anesthetics are among the most commonly employed drugs in medi-cine. Anyone who has ever had dental work or stitches for a deep cut knows what pain-eliminating lifesavers these drugs are. At the same time they are also responsible for a variety of adverse nonimmunologic reactions, such as central nervous system and cardiac toxicities, and for a variety of presumed allergic problems, including contact dermatitis, hives, giant hives, and anaphylaxis. Problems arise when the physician is asked to help the surgeon or dentist choose an alternative local anesthetic for a patient who has a history of an allergy to a particular local anesthetic.

For practical purposes, local anesthetics can be divided into two main classes. Group I includes such familiar anesthetics as benzocaine (found in many topical anti-itch and antisunburn preparations), tetracaine, and procaine (**Novocain**). Group II includes lidocaine (**Xylocaine**, which is probably the most universally used injectable local anesthetic today), mepivicaine, cyclomethycaine, and dibucaine. If you are allergic to one member of a group, you are likely to be allergic to other members of the same group. Fortunately, however, there is little cross-allergenicity: If you are allergic to **Novocain** from Group I, your dentist may substitute lidocaine (**Xylocaine**) from Group II without fear of provoking cross-allergy.

Occasionally, skin testing, using prick and intradermal administration of increasing concentrations, may be needed to determine a person's allergic status to local anesthetics. To accomplish this, the individual is challenged by subcutaneous administration (injections into the fat) of increasing doses of the suspected allergen to see if there is evidence of local reaction. As with penicillin testing, skin testing with anesthetics must be performed under strict medical supervision.

DIAGNOSIS

Since there are few truly helpful laboratory tests for drug allergy, the history of the events surrounding the onset of a particular drug reaction is the single most important step used by doctors to determine the diagnosis. Most often the problem confronting your doctor is whether your symptoms are those related to a drug or to an infectious germ. If you develop allergy symptoms while taking several drugs for different conditions, pinpointing the precise cause becomes that much more complicated. But even when the cause has been narrowed to a specific drug, the reaction may not necessarily be the result of allergy to the active ingredient. Instead, it may be to one or more of the additives, which may not even be listed on the package label or package insert.

Laboratory Tests

Laboratory testing is less than helpful in the workup of most drug reactions. For one thing, the actual drug is seldom the direct cause of the problem. For another, we often do not know which of its breakdown byproducts or metabolites (with the notable exception of penicillin)is the problem or with which body proteins the drug may combine in order to trigger allergic symptoms. Although by no means diagnostic or specific, finding an elevated count of eosinophils (a special kind of white blood cell) in a routine blood test helps support a suspected diagnosis of drug allergy.

Direct skin testing to detect immediate hypersensitivity (IgE) drug allergies has so far proven consistently valuable for diagnosing only penicillin, insulin, and local anesthetic allergies. Likewise, the RAST has also to date proven of limited usefulness to physicians. In some cases of suspected drug-allergy-induced anemias or bleeding disorders, certain specialized blood tests have been helpful for establishing the diagnosis.

Patch testing, by contrast, has been proven invaluable in the workup of suspected cases of contact dermatitis or photoallergic dermatitis. In patch testing, tiny amounts of presumed allergens are placed against the skin under Band-Aid-like patches in an attempt to reproduce the allergic symptoms at the test site (see Appendix A). Photoallergy testing requires the additional step of exposing the test sites to ultraviolet A radiation in an effort to provoke the allergic response.

All things considered, the only conclusive way to prove that any drug is the cause of an allergic problem is to rechallenge the individual with the same drug after it has been discontinued and after all prior symptoms have cleared. Such a therapeutic (or drug) challenge, as doctors call it, is generally contemplated only when the particular medication in question is the only drug or is by far the best drug available to treat a condition.

In general, if the allergic symptoms are mild—just itching, for example—the risk of a therapeutic challenge is small. However, when airway constriction, falling blood pressure, or shock has occurred previously, the risk is great, and therefore the test should be done under the strictest medical supervision, if at all. Drug challenges are the only definitive means for confirming allergy to aspirin or radio-contrast media (materials that are commonly used in many types of diagnostic X-ray examinations). They are also an excellent means of determining allergies to local anesthetics.

PREVENTION

By far the best method of preventing drug allergies is to take as few medications as you can and as infrequently as you can. This means not running to the medicine cabinet and popping a few antibiotic tablets that have been lying around from the last illness to treat some current problem without first consulting your doctor. Besides, taking antibiotics (which work only against bacteria anyway) in order to treat your virus cold or flu is a bad practice. All you really accomplish by this is increasing your chances of becoming unnecessarily sensitized to medications that you may really need someday for a serious illness. And while both erythromycin and tetracycline, two of the most frequently used broad-spectrum antibiotics, possess a low potential for provoking allergies, they should still not be used indiscriminately in order to reduce any risk of unnecessary sensitization.

Common sense likewise dictates that should you experience any symptoms, particularly breathing problems, hives, itching, or any other kinds of rashes after taking a certain drug, you should stop it at once and consult your doctor. Leave it to your physician to determine whether your problems are truly allergic in nature and whether an alternative therapy should be instituted.

Another good tip is to avoid medications that provide "shotgun" treatments for certain conditions. For example, many OTC cold preparations contain antiallergy, anticongestion, anticough, and antifever ingredients. If you have a fever and a hacking cough, you are better off taking a separate antipyretic (fever reducer) such as acetaminophen (such as **Tylenol**) and an anticough syrup containing dextromethorphan (such as **Benylin DM**) than a combination preparation that contains a host of additional ingredients for symptoms you don't have. By doing so you are better able to regulate the individual dosage of the drugs you need rather than taking the fixed amounts contained in the combination preparation (which may be either too much or too little for your specific needs).

Wearing a Medic Alert bracelet or necklace is another valuable preventive measure, especially for those who have experienced a life-threatening reaction to a common drug such as penicillin, sulfa, or aspirin. (The Medic Alert bracelet or necklace is also a good idea for insulin-dependent diabetics, severe asthmatics, and persons who have experienced life-threatening reactions to bee and wasp stings.) Looking very much like a dog tag, these necklaces and bracelets provide physicians and other emergency personnel with vital medical information in the event that you are unable to do so. (The address of Medic Alert, a nonprofit foundation, is P.O. Box 1009, Turlock, California 95380.)

TREATMENT

The best treatment for any suspected allergic reaction to a medication is the commonsense measure of stopping the drug at once. Severe reactions often require emergency treatment with epinephrine (**Adrenalin**), antihistamines, and systemic corticosteroid medications to suppress symptoms. Mild skin reactions can frequently be treated with bland, soothing hypoallergenic emollients alone. More severe reactions may require topical corticosteroid creams or lotions. Finally, OTC anti-itch creams containing either the topical anesthetic benzocaine or the antihistamine diphenhydramine should be avoided because these agents have been associated with a high risk of provoking allergic contact dermatitis in a fair proportion of people. In any event, if you have a specific question about any drug you are taking or applying, you should consult with your doctor or pharmacist promptly.

CHAPTER EIGHT

ITCHING, SCRATCHING, AND RASHING: OH, THOSE MISERABLE SKIN ALLERGIES

W│hile some people may view skin conditions as nothing more than annoyances or trivial problems, for many others they are causes of significant distress and may even compromise their life-styles. Many complaints of itching or rashing are related to allergenic substances that are applied to or come in contact with the skin either at home or in the workplace. Regarding the latter, the National Institute for Occupational Safety and Health (NIOSH) maintains that widespread, debilitating work-related skin disorders are the most pervasive current occupational health problem in the United States, accounting for more than one-third of all work-related health problems. Since occurrences in the home go unreported, one can only speculate on the extent of the problem there, but it is likely to be quite widespread and significantly distressing as well.

CONTACT DERMATITIS

Before discussing the subject of allergic contact skin allergy, or *allergic contact dermatitis*, as dermatologists call it, you need to understand the essential difference between an irritant contact dermatitis and an allergic contact dermatitis. Occasionally the signs and symptoms of each are so similar that even your doctor may find it difficult to distinguish between the two.

Irritant Contact Dermatitis

Not every skin rash stemming from contact with a certain chemical substance is an allergy. In fact, the vast majority of reactions, about 90 percent, that result from direct skin contact are *nonimmunologic* or irritant reactions and for that reason merit inclusion in any discussion of contact-induced skin eruptions. Strictly defined, irritant contact dermatitis is any form of toxic skin reaction due to direct skin contact with either harsh or caustic chemicals or other environmental agents found in the home or workplace. But unlike allergic reactions, in which only predisposed ("previously sensitized") individuals are at risk, irritant reactions, particularly those caused by strong irritants, can happen to anyone who is exposed to the irritating substance. In other words, direct contact with concentrated sulfuric acid would be expected to irritate or burn anyone's hands severely, not just some people's.

Common irritants include paints and solvents (such as alcohol, acetone, turpentine, and carbon tetrachloride); surfactants (soaps, detergents, and emulsifying agents); drying agents (astringents, toners, clarifying lotions, and others); abrasives (such as particle-containing soaps and facial masks); acids (such as battery acid and acid-containing cosmetics), alkalis (such as household lye and drain cleaners); wood preservatives; cement; lime; oils and tars; enzymes (either naturally occurring or synthetic chemicals used to speed up chemical or metabolic reactions); and certain hypertonic (highly concentrated) solutions. Even plastics and some metals may cause irritant contact dermatitis.

As a group, soaps—which function to permit normally water-repellent grease and grime to be rinsed away by plain water—are one of the most common kinds of irritants because they also compromise the skin's barrier function by removing the natural oils necessary for maintaining the integrity of the upper layers. Repetitive use (especially of pure alkaline soaps or abrasive cleansers) opens the way to abnormal skin water loss and chapping. In addition, traces of soap residue that are often left on the skin after washing can themselves further irritate the skin, especially when coupled with wetness or perspiration. Many people are affected in this way.

When it comes to irritant reactions to weaker agents than soaps, there seem to be individual differences in tolerance to irritation. This is possibly due to inherited variations in the thinness of the upper layers of the skin or to differences in amounts of natural surface oils. As a rule, thick-skinned and oily-skinned persons tend to be more resistant to irritation.

The specific site of exposure as well as environmental factors also play a role in this condition. For example, the thin, more permeable skin of the eyelid, the face, and the genitals are far more likely to react to irritants than the thicker skin of the extremities, trunk, or buttocks. In general, high humidity tends to increase the possibility of irritation because moisture enhances the penetration of irritants. And at the other extreme, very low humidity, by drying and chapping the skin, can also promote irritant reactions.

Despite the existence of myths to the contrary, there seem to be no clear-cut racial, sexual, or age barriers as to who is most likely to suffer irritant reactions. For example, medical science has debunked the common myth that white skin is more prone to irritation than black skin. In fact, current research suggests that the reverse may even be true. Similarly, investigations have questioned the notion that women are more susceptible than men. While such reactions are indeed more common in women, many believe this reflects their greater overall exposure to potential irritants (by way of cosmetics and household cleaning products) than it does to any inherent gender predisposition. Finally, while factors such as thinner skin and decreased natural oil gland secretion would lead one to predict that elderly skin is more easily irritated than younger skin, this also is not necessarily the case. When it comes to resistance or susceptibility to irritant reactions, mature skin seems to fare about as well as younger skin.

Signs and Symptoms

As a rule, the signs and symptoms of irritant dermatitis depend on the potency of the irritant and the length of time it is in contact with the skin. Reactions to strong agents may begin within minutes of the very first exposure, while reactions to milder irritants may appear within weeks or even months of repeated exposure. Mild reactions generally give rise to dryness and cracking, which are often observed on hands and forearms. Brisker reactions may run the gamut from redness and swelling to blisters, pustules, fissures (superficial splitting of the skin), and even ulcers (deep splits in the skin). Most people with irritant contact dermatitis complain of some combination of stinging, itching, burning, or pain.

Diagnosis

For the physician, the patient's history is by far the most useful diagnostic aid to date. In many cases it is a fairly straightforward matter to recognize the problem and pinpoint the culprit irritant when only a single, very potent agent is suspected. For example, if a person develops a severe rash on his hands thirty minutes after prolonged, ungloved contact with turpentine-soaked brushes, the reaction is likely to be an irritant dermatitis to turpentine.

On the other hand, when there has been exposure to a number of differing, weaker irritants over an extended period of time, it can be much more challenging to determine the actual troublemaker(s). Moreover, especially in the case of weak irritants, it may also be difficult to distinguish an irritant reaction from a true allergic contact allergy.

Patch tests (see Appendix A), in which small amounts of suspected materials are placed in contact with the skin, can occasionally be helpful in confirming suspected irritants (although, as we've discussed, they are far more useful for determining contact allergens). One problem is the obvious risk of provoking an intense irritation or

burn at the test site. A second difficulty involves the occasional problem of distinguishing a positive irritant patch test reaction to a weak
irritant from an allergic one. In general, irritant patch test reactions
appear and disappear quickly and tend to be confined to the area of
direct contact. Allergic reactions, by contrast, take longer to develop,
last longer, and spread beyond the patch site to the surrounding skin.
Nevertheless, telling the two apart is not always easy, and doctors carefully evaluate the results of the patch tests in terms of the patient's
history before drawing any conclusions.

Prevention and Treatment

Avoiding contact with a suspected irritant altogether is by far the
best form of prevention. When you can't completely avoid contact,
you should at least use protective clothing, such as gloves, aprons,
and so forth, whenever possible. Rather than purchasing the familiar
cotton-lined latex gloves, you would do better to purchase an individual pair of thick vinyl outer gloves as well as several pairs of pure
cotton undergloves. Although this may seem somewhat inconve-
nient, it is far better for the skin. For one thing, vinyl is less allergenic
than latex. For another, since it is virtually impossible to adequately
clean the cotton linings of the ordinary combination gloves, you may
actually experience irritation from the perspiration and dirt buildup
that develops inside them after several uses. It is a simple matter,
however, to launder the cotton linings if you wear separate cotton
undergloves. You can purchase vinyl and cotton gloves at surgical
supply stores, or you may order them directly from specialty companies such as Allerderm Laboratories, Box 931, Mill Valley, California
94942. If you use the gloves for extended periods of time, you should
change the cotton undergloves frequently—about every twenty
minutes—to reduce the likelihood of irritation from perspiration
buildup.

Barrier creams are another method of reducing direct contact with irritants. They are not nearly as protective as gloves, but many of these products are capable of providing a high measure of protection for up to four hours, even against certain acids and corrosives. Examples of effective barrier creams include **Wonder Glove, Dermaffin**, and **Dermashield**. For optimal protection, however, I advise the use of barrier creams in addition to protective gloves. Since dry skin and chapping generally make skin more susceptible to irritations of all kinds, I also suggest that you liberally apply an all-purpose, fragrance-free moisturizer containing both occlusive and humectant ingredients such as **Curel** routinely after you wash or shower. And for persons with exceptionally dry skin, I generally recommend **Lac-Hydrin** lotion, a potent, prescription-only moisturizer that contains lactic acid.

Several other commonsense measures to reduce unnecessary irritation include avoiding hot water, employing tongs to handle wet laundry, switching to disposable diapers, using a brush to wash dishes, or, better still, purchasing an automatic dishwasher. Direct handling of raw meat and poultry as well as raw vegetables, particularly tomatoes, potatoes, and citrus fruits, should be avoided as much as possible. In addition, to minimize having your hands in water continuously all day, try to arrange your wet-work chores so they are all done at one time during the day. In other words, collect all the dishes from several courses and wash them together rather than a few at a time throughout the meal. As a group, household chores can take such a toll on your skin, particularly the hands, that housework-related irritant contact dermatitis is often called "housewife's eczema" or "housewife's hands."

Using mild, synthetic detergent cleansers rather than true soaps, abrasive cleansers, or deodorant soaps for routine cleansing can also reduce the likelihood of irritation. You should look for liquid or bar cleansers that are labeled for sensitive skin. Preferably, these should also be fragrance-free and hypoallergenic (for example, there is **Oil of Olay Sensitive Skin Bath Bar**). Finally, avoid abrasive scrub brushes, polyester sponges, or even washcloths since they tend to overly rub and abrade the skin, making irritation more likely.

ALLERGIC CONTACT DERMATITIS

Although much less common than irritant dermatitis, allergic contact dermatitis is still an important source of problems for many people. As the name suggests, this type of reaction is not a simple matter of direct irritation but is a true allergic condition mediated by the skin's complex immune system. While allergic contact dermatitis can be produced by just about any substance, some agents are more likely to trigger it than others. Poison ivy dermatitis, nickel allergy, and latex allergy are three well-known examples of allergic contact sensitivity that can serve to illustrate many of the main aspects of allergic contact skin conditions.

Poison Ivy Dermatitis

The term poison ivy is misleading. The milky saplike resin, called a *catechol*, that is responsible for the rash of this condition and that of its relatives, poison sumac and poison oak, is not a poison at all but a true allergen. In the United States, the overall incidence of allergy to the poison ivy family of plants is estimated to be between 50 percent and 75 percent of the population.

Sensitization (the immunologic reactions that establish allergy) generally requires a week to two weeks. While some people become allergic to these plants following their first exposure to the resin, many others do not. In fact, it often takes numerous exposures before the allergy develops. However, once sensitization is complete, subsequent reexposures to the poison ivy resin generally result in symptoms in a much briefer period, usually somewhere between five and seventy-two hours after contact.

The extent and severity of poison ivy reactions depend in large measure on how much of your skin comes in contact with the resin, how much is deposited on the skin, and how innately sensitive you are to it. In other words, the more allergic to poison ivy you are and the more of the sap you get on you, the worse your reaction will be. Typical symptoms consist of intense redness, swelling, and blistering at the sites of contact. Occasionally, the allergic reaction can be quite severe and debilitating. Because the poison ivy vines or shrubs tend to brush up against you as you pass, the blisters and the rash are typically distributed in a streaklike or linelike fashion along the skin.

Patients with poison ivy invariably become concerned about spreading their condition to others. Since the reaction is an allergy, not an infection, the concern is happily unfounded. You cannot spread your allergy to someone else, not even if they come in direct contact with the blister fluid itself. Should the blisters open, however, the possibility of secondary bacterial infection increases, and you need to be especially careful at that point because the infection (not the allergy) can be spread to others.

Prevention is the best form of treatment for poison ivy dermatitis. This means wearing protective clothing—gloves, long-sleeved shirts, and long pants, for example—when gardening or hiking. Several recently introduced barrier creams can also be useful. These include **Stokogard, Hollister Moisture Barrier**, and **Hydropel**. In one study, the allergic reaction to plant resins was blunted more than 50 percent by the prophylactic use of these agents. Nevertheless, avoidance and the use of protective clothing remain the best forms of prevention.

When inadvertent contact with the plant is made, the skin should be cleansed thoroughly with soap and water or, better still, cleansed with plain rubbing alcohol to dissolve the resin. This is most effective when done within the first fifteen minutes after exposure, before skin binding by the resin is complete. After that time, a topical preparation such as **Calamine lotion** or **Sarna lotion** may be tried to promote drying of the lesions and to decrease itching. In many cases these simple measures will suffice.

More severe or widespread reactions frequently require the use of topical corticosteroid antiinflammatory agents, which are some of the most widely used preparations in dermatology today and the mainstays of dermatitis therapy. Depending on the severity of the condition, your doctor may prescribe a high-, medium- or low-potency variety in a lotion, gel, cream, or ointment formulation. In most cases topical corticosteroids are applied once or twice daily, and you can generally anticipate complete relief from the rash and itching within a few days. Topical steroids are usually discontinued once the symptoms have cleared, but some physicians may advise continuing them for a little while longer to reduce the small (but real) possibility of a rebound flare-up of the problem. **Ultravate**, **Temovate**, and **Diprolene** are brand-name examples of super-high-potency topical steroids, and **Aclovate**, **Elocon**, **Locoid**, and **Hytone** are examples of intermediate- and low-strength formulations.

Occasionally, poison ivy may be so severe that your doctor will prescribe an oral corticosteroid preparation such as prednisone or **Decadron** to bring your symptoms under control. These, too, in decreasing doses, may be continued for a week or two following the clearing of the symptoms to prevent relapse. Finally, when bacteria have invaded, a topical or oral antibiotic may also be prescribed to clear the infection and prevent its spread.

Nickel Dermatitis

Dealing with an allergy to nickel can be a difficult problem; so many common items contain the metal that it is hard for nickel-sensitive persons to avoid it. It is found in such things as coins, medallions, scissors, thimbles, needles, zippers, buckles, garters, clips, hairpins, curlers, pens, and costume jewelry. It is also hidden in stainless-steel materials, products made of alnico, Ticonium, and Invar, and chrome-plated items. Even expensive gold jewelry is alloyed with nickel to give it strength.

As with all allergic contact dermatitis reactions, the rash of nickel allergy appears at the points of contact and often is the size and shape of the metal object that provoked it. For example, identification tag and necklace reactions typically involve the upper chest and back; hairpin, curler, and eyeglass reactions, the scalp and face; coin and scissor allergies, the fingers; and earrings, the earlobes. Regardless of what item is the culprit, however, nickel allergies typically appear as itchy, red, scaly rashes within hours of contact.

As in the case of poison ivy rashes, prevention is the best form of therapy, and all known nickel-containing items should be avoided as much as possible. Moreover, since moisture and sweating increase the likelihood of nickel rashes in susceptible persons, the frequent dusting of talcum powder at areas of contact, such as under watches, can be helpful in reducing possible reactions. And if you don't want to give up wearing jewelry altogether, special hypoallergenic surgical stainless-steel and sterling silver jewelry is available. Alternatively, you may try covering your favorite earrings with a thick layer of lacquer to prevent direct contact with the nickel.

Once you know for sure that you are allergic to nickel, a testing product known as the **SpotTest** kit, which contains the chemical *dimethylglyoxime*, may be used to test household items and jewelry for the presence of nickel. A small amount of the clear liquid testing solution is applied with a cotton swab to the item to be tested. If the object contains nickel, a pink or red color appears. Each kit is usually good for about two hundred tests.

Topical corticosteroids are the treatment of choice for severe, acute, or chronic nickel rashes.

Latex Rubber Dermatitis

With the increasing use of condoms to prevent the spread of AIDS and other sexually transmissible diseases and with the increased use of latex surgical gloves for the routine physical examinations of patients, there has been an alarming rise in the incidence of allergic reactions to latex rubber. In other words, because of increased exposure to latex products, more people are becoming allergic to it than ever before.

At present between 1 percent and 2 percent of the population is allergic to latex rubber, and as many as 10 percent of all health-care workers (that is, physicians, dentists, nurses, and so forth) are now latex-sensitized. Allergic contact rashes on the hands are the most common manifestation, but, though rare, shock and even death from immediate hypersensitive allergy have been reported. By itself, natural rubber is almost never a sensitizer; rather, the culprits are the many different chemicals that go in to the vulcanization and manufacture of rubber products. These include residual latex proteins, mercaptobenzothiazole (MBT), and thiurams.

Fortunately, while other substitutes are being actively sought, a number of alternatives to latex have been available for some time. For example, garments containing spandex, a synthetic elastic fiber, have been around for a number of years and can be recognized by the manufacturer's names. And industrial-strength synthetic rubber gloves made of neoprene have also been available for a while.

Likewise, sexually active persons with latex allergies may currently turn to styrene or polymer condoms for effective contraception and infection control. While the use of natural, skin-type condoms (made from sheep's intestine) would seem like a logical alternative when one partner, or both partners, is latex-sensitive, such condoms unfortunately do not provide adequate protection against transmissible sexual diseases. For the moment, then, the use of two types of condoms has been suggested in order to minimize allergic problems while ensuring both adequate contraception and disease prevention. If the sexually receptive individual is latex-allergic, the partner may first apply a latex condom and then a natural condom over it before insertion. If the situation is reversed, however, and the user is allergic to latex, then the natural condom should be applied first and the latex one over it to prevent direct contact with his skin. Looking to the not-too-distant future, a woman's condom made of polyurethane plastic, which at this time is still under investigation by the Federal Drug Administration, will no doubt be welcomed by latex-sensitive couples.

Fortunately, health-care workers may also choose from several alternatives. To avoid the problem entirely, many choose to use disposable vinyl gloves whenever possible because they contain no rubber derivatives at all. But when greater dexterity is required, they may select **Elastryn**, a specially designed hypoallergic glove made of nonvulcanized rubber. Surgeons who require sterile, anatomically fit gloves may purchase products made of tactylon, a nonlatex, nonvulcanized synthetic copolymer (**Tactyl**) or those made from a group of fancy-sounding substances known as accelerated antibiodioxidants (specifically, **Neolon** and **Dermaprene**). **Biogel gloves**, a newcomer to the medical marketplace, claims to have virtually undetectable levels of allergenic latex proteins and extremely low levels of potentially allergenic rubber accelerators in both its sterile and nonsterile glove lines.

Keep in mind that not every allergy to rubber products is related to the latex protein itself. Allergy to examination gloves, for example, may be due to the powders or starches that coat the inside of them to absorb perspiration and to facilitate application and removal. In the case of condoms, allergies may be due to the preservatives in the wet jellies used to coat the lubricated varieties or, less commonly, to the silicone-based lubricants used in the dry varieties. If this is the case, simply changing the type of product you use may end the problem.

When suspected, dermatologists can test for latex allergy through a "use" test. In this test, a rubber glove or just the finger portions are worn on damp hands for between fifteen and thirty minutes and are then checked for the development of a rash. Alternatively, or in addition, the physician may cut a small square of latex and apply it as a patch test directly to the back or inner arm and evaluate it for allergic changes in forty-eight to seventy-two hours.

For most cases of rubber-induced rashes, treatment consists of a short course of topical steroid creams. Though rare, oral steroids may be needed to suppress the inflammation.

Much of what has just been said about poison ivy, nickel allergy, and latex contact allergy applies equally to all the many other substances found in your home or workplace that may trigger contact allergies. In order of frequency, these include: *neomycin*, which is found in many OTC topical antibiotic preparations; *thimerosal*, which is a preservative found in many topical and ophthalmic preparations such as contact lens solutions; *formaldehyde*, which is encountered in permanent press clothing and many other industrial products; *quarternium 15*, which is a common preservative ingredient and a formaldehyde-releasing chemical that is used widely in industry; *paraphenylenediamine*, which is the most common hair dye agent in use today; *balsam of Peru*, which is a popular fragrance; and *cinnamic alcohol*, which is a common aromatic and flavoring ingredient. Other well-known culprits may be found in certain cosmetics (see Chapter 9), clothing (wool, synthetic fibers, dyes, and leather), many kinds of household items (such as detergents, disinfectants, bleaches, polishes, and waxes), and numerous workplace items (cements, glues, plastics, and paints).

In the past few years, the use of skin patches for the delivery of medication, such as estrogen for menopausal symptoms and scopolamine for motion sickness, have become increasingly popular. At the same time, such *transdermal delivery systems*, as they are known medically, have also become responsible for a growing number of instances of allergic contact dermatitis. Transdermal clonidine, an antihypertensive agent, has so far accounted for the majority of allergic contact reactions. Curiously, most people who are unable to tolerate the clonidine patches are able to take the medication orally without any problem.

In most cases of allergic contact dermatitis, the history and the location of the condition provide strong clues to the diagnosis. As part of the workup, your doctor will usually question you in detail about your home routines, occupational activities, and hobbies, exploring possible exposure to cosmetics, plants, and topical medications, both OTC and physician-prescribed.

When allergic contact dermatitis is strongly suspected but no specific agent can be pinpointed definitively as the troublemaker, your doctor may suggest patch-testing on normal skin with a *screening battery* of allergens. A standard screening battery contains many of the allergens known to be used in the home and in industry. Once a particular allergen is identified by this method, the doctor can provide you with a list of specific products and items to avoid.

Photoallergic Contact Dermatitis

Because of its unique aspects, photoallergic contact dermatitis deserves special mention. In this condition, the sun's ultraviolet rays convert an otherwise harmless chemical into an allergen, and persons with photocontact allergies generally show up at the dermatologist's office complaining that they have developed an "allergy to the sun." It is, however, an allergy to a specific chemical substance applied to the skin that has been promoted by the sun; by themselves, neither the sun nor the chemical is usually capable of provoking the dermatitis. Photocontact allergens include topical antibacterials, such as the halogenated salicylanalides, cosmetics, fragrances, and even sunscreen ingredients.

Confirming a diagnosis of photoallergic contact dermatitis requires the same steps as those involved in diagnosing ordinary allergic contact dermatitis, with one major exception: Instead of employing simple patch tests to isolate the allergen(s), *photopatch tests* must be performed. The patches of test materials are usually removed somewhere between one and three days after they are applied, and then the skin sites underneath are irradiated briefly with ultraviolet A (UVA) light. Following this, they are covered once again and then examined two days later for the presence of dermatitis (see Appendix A).

As in the case of ordinary contact allergies, simply discontinuing the use of the offending substance will put an end to the problem. When this is not possible, the use of high SPF sunscreen or sunblock agents is advisable. But if the problem happens to be the sunscreen itself, a suitable substitute must be sought. For example, if you are found to be allergic to PABA or PABA derivatives, which are very common sunscreen agents, you should look for non-PABA-containing sunscreens, of which quite a number are currently available. If you still have a problem, you might try one of the several chemical-free sunblock agents that contain miconized titanium dioxide, such as **Neutrogena's Chemical-Free Sunblocker.**

Once under way, severe photoallergic reactions need to be quieted with topical corticosteroid creams, oral antihistamines, and short courses of oral corticosteroids.

Contact Urticaria

Like contact dermatitis, contact urticaria, or hives, which result from the dilation of the small blood vessels in the skin and leakage of fluid into the surrounding tissue, may be triggered by direct contact with allergenic substances or, more commonly, through direct contact with various irritating agents. Sometimes called welts or wheals, hives are pinkish swellings of the skin and mucous membranes that are usually very itchy and generally last no more than twenty-four hours, often fading somewhere up to six hours after first developing. Ordinary hives range in size from half an inch to twelve inches or more in diameter. Extremely large, swollen hives are called *angioedema* and may extend the length of an entire extremity or swell the entire face.

Despite the fact that all the chemical mediators responsible for contact urticaria have yet to be identified, histamine is believed to play a major role in the production of the itching, redness, and swelling seen in this condition. In nonallergic cases of contact urticaria, the provocative agent somehow induces the direct release of histamine (and other agents) from mast cells and basophils. IgE, the same antibody involved in triggering attacks of asthma and allergic rhinitis, is believed to be responsible for doing so in allergic cases.

As in the case of irritant contact dermatitis, irritant (or nonimmunologic) contact urticaria may be triggered by a wide variety of substances. Well-known triggers of nonallergic contact urticaria include chemicals naturally found in certain foods, fragrances, flavorings, colorings, and preservatives, as well as additives in soaps, shampoos, toothpastes, and so forth. Specific troublemakers include benzoic acid, sodium benzoate, sorbic acid, cinnamic aldehyde, balsam of Peru, acetic acid, butyric acid, and various alcohols.

While the eruption of allergic contact urticaria looks very much like its nonallergic counterpart, a number of clues help your doctor distinguish between the two. For one thing, individuals with the allergic variety demonstrate an allergy to a particular substance that affects only a small percentage of the population at large. Irritants, by contrast, tend to provoke symptoms in the majority of people. In addition, truly allergic persons generally give a history of previous exposure to the presumed allergen sometime in the past that was not followed by the onset of any symptoms. Those with nonallergic rashes usually recall the onset of the problem the very first time they came in contact with the particular substance. And finally, allergic individuals typically report a pattern of worsening symptoms after each episode of contact, while those with irritant urticaria do not.

The list of potential contact urticaria allergens is very long. Some of the more important ones that have been associated with the reaction include bacitracin, benzoyl peroxide, lindane, menthol, neomycin, nickel, parabens, sunscreens, plastic additives, henna, hair sprays, nail polish, perfumes, birch and teak woods, milk, spices, eggs, meats, flour, and even seminal fluid.

The diagnosis of either variety of contact urticaria rests mostly on the history. Blood testing is rarely helpful, but open patch tests have proven useful in some cases related to cosmetics. In these tests a tiny amount of each test material is applied with a glass rod to a half-inch-square area of skin on the hairless part of the forearm. After thirty minutes the sites are checked for the onset of tingling, itching, redness, and hiving. Prick tests, in which small amounts of suspected materials are injected into the skin, are rarely used nowadays because of the potential risk of provoking severe and even life-threatening reactions.

Naturally, avoiding the offending substance is the best form of treatment for all forms of contact urticaria. Acute attacks are usually treated with topical corticosteroid creams and oral antihistamines. More severe attacks may require a short course of an oral corticosteroid, such as prednisone, **Medrol**, or **Decadron**.

Atopic Dermatitis

Atopic dermatitis, often called atopic eczema or simply eczema, is a common condition affecting approximately 3 percent of the American population of all ages, and about 10 percent of all younger people between infancy and early adulthood. It eventually disappears in all but about 3 percent of people. In 70 percent to 80 percent of cases, there is a family history of one or more of the following allergic conditions: asthma, hay fever (or allergic rhinitis), hives, and atopic dermatitis. This suggests a family trait or genetic predisposition for the development of this problem.

To date there is still no conclusive proof that atopic dermatitis is an allergic disorder, but a fairly substantial amount of indirect evidence suggests that allergy plays a role, at least in some cases. For example, in about 10 percent of children, the disease can be triggered or worsened by allergic reactions to certain foods. Eggs, fish, milk, peanuts, soy, and wheat are common allergic triggers. Within as short a time as half an hour after consuming these foods, susceptible individuals may experience redness and itching. Merely stopping the culprit food often leads to complete clearing. Additionally, the link already noted between atopic eczema and asthma, hay fever, and hives is another strong piece of indirect evidence for an underlying allergic basis. Likewise, allergies to house dust and house dust mites have also been implicated in some cases. And finally, some researchers have recently found greater amounts of IgE antibodies (the so-called allergy antibodies) bound to the cells within the upper and middle layers of the skin of atopic individuals as compared with the skin of non-eczema-prone persons.

Nevertheless, nonallergic mechanisms are also believed to play a significant role in many cases. Dry skin, for example, often precipitates a flare-up of atopic dermatitis and is particularly troublesome during the wintertime due to the wet, chapping conditions of the outdoors and the drying condition of indoor heating. Summertime, too, has its difficulties because of the artificially lowered humidity from air-conditioning and the excessive dryness and irritation caused by the chlorine in swimming pools. And at any time of the year atopic dermatitis may be aggravated by the overzealous use of strong soaps and hot water. Finally, nervous tension and physical illnesses—major ones as well as minor ones such as colds, fevers, sore throats, and ear infections—are other well-known causes of flare-ups.

Diagnosis

The rash of atopic dermatitis is more likely to develop on the exposed areas of the skin, presumably because of the increased likelihood of chapping, drying, and environmental contact at these sites. In severe cases, however, the rash may occur anywhere on the body or even cover the entire skin surface. In young adults it typically involves the face, the folds of the elbows, and the backs of the knees, but it spares the groin. Affected patches are dry, scaly, reddish, and intensely and unrelentingly itchy (one of the hallmarks of the disorder). In chronic (persistent) cases, the involved areas eventually become lackluster, thickened, and brownish and are frequently covered with scratch marks and crusts.

In most instances dermatologists are able to diagnose atopic dermatitis fairly easily. It is strongly suggested in anyone with eczema who has a family and/or a personal history of asthma, allergic rhinitis, and hives. While there are no definitive tests for the condition, the finding of elevated blood IgE levels in someone with the skin manifestations of eczema is considered an additional support for the diagnosis.

Prevention

Given what has been said, susceptible individuals should take every precaution against overdrying and overchapping their skin. This means limiting showers to no more than three minutes at a time and using tepid rather than hot water. It is advisable to avoid washcloths and polyester scrub sponges, which unnecessarily abrade the skin, and to use mild synthetic detergent cleansers, as described above, instead of soaps that are pure alkaline, degreasing, deodorant, or abrasive. For those who absolutely cannot give up that nice, long, luxurious soak in the bathtub, I recommend the use of **Alpha-Keri Bath Oil** or **Actibath Carbonated Tablets**; they can be added to the bath water to offset some of the dryness. Whenever possible, choose garments made of pure cotton, especially intimate apparel, and select loose-fitting clothing rather than tight, constricting garments that rub the skin. Wool or other scratchy materials should be avoided since they can be especially irritating. In addition, wearing appropriate weather-protective clothing in the wintertime, getting plenty of rest, and trying to avoid colds also makes good sense under the circumstances.

Special effort must be made to protect the skin from drying. Shallow pans of water placed near radiators around the house or the use of cold air humidifiers are useful measures for reducing household dryness. If you enjoy chlorine swimming (beach swimming is generally better for the skin), you should coat yourself liberally with a hypoallergenic, all-purpose moisturizer before entering the water and once again immediately after rinsing off in the shower after swimming. For outdoor swimming, a moisturizing sunscreen such as **Oil of Olay Daily UV Protectant** is a reasonable choice. If additional moisture is needed, you might discuss with your doctor the use of the prescription-strength moisturizing lotion **Lac-Hydrin** for routine use and before and after swimming.

If a food allergy is believed to be contributing to the problem, your doctor may recommend a two-week trial of a nutritionally sound elimination diet, consisting of chicken (baked or broiled), lamb, rice, yams, broccoli, cauliflower, apples, and pears (cooked or canned), salt, and water. If improvement is seen during this time, the link to some food allergy is established. Thereafter, to determine the specific food culprit by looking for a flare-up, a new food group is usually reintroduced into your diet every four days. Breads, pastas, and cereals are generally added first, and other food groups are subsequently added slowly until the culprit foods are eventually discovered. The method may seem to be a long-drawn-out affair, but in the end it is more reliable than skin testing, which has a notoriously high rate of misleading results in cases of atopic dermatitis.

Treatment

Unfortunately, we are still unable to cure atopic dermatitis. Nevertheless, your dermatologist can prescribe a variety of simple measures and medications that will substantially alleviate your symptoms and clear up the rash. As in the case of other forms of eczema, the therapy for moderate and severe atopic dermatitis generally includes the prescription of topical corticosteroid creams alone or combined with oral antihistamines and, occasionally, brief courses of oral corticosteroids.

The use of topical steroids, especially high-potency agents, in atopic dermatitis, which is a long-term problem that may require years of therapy, demands a strong word of caution. While they may look like ordinary cold cream or petroleum jelly when applied to your skin, topical steroids should be used only under the strict supervision of a physician to prevent complications. If they are used on a daily basis for several weeks, the more potent classes in particular may cause irreversible, premature thinning of the skin, increased fragility, the development of "broken" blood vessels, skin pigment loss, and stretch marks. Used cautiously under a doctor's supervision, however, they are wonderful, neat preparations that offer sufferers welcome rapid relief.

Finally, in order to wean eczema patients from topical steroids once the rash has cleared and as part of a subsequent maintenance program to reduce the likelihood and severity of recurrences, I have found that, once again, **Lac-Hydrin** lotion is especially useful. Besides its value as a moisturizer, recent evidence suggests that it may have a protective effect against the skin-thinning effects of topical steroids when its use is alternated with the application of the steroid each day. Active research into atopic dermatitis promises still better and more specific therapies in the future.

CHAPTER NINE

WHEN MAKEUP MAKES TROUBLE: SENSITIVE SKIN AND COSMETIC ALLERGIES

SENSITIVE SKIN

D oes the following sound familiar to you? "I just don't know what to do for my skin anymore. I'm so disgusted! I've tried just about everything I can think of—at least twenty different makeups and even products labeled hypoallergenic—but they all irritate me! I've always had sensitive skin, even when I was a teenager, but isn't there something I can use that won't cause problems?"

"Sensitive skin" is one of the most frequent laments of new patients who come to my office. But one of the biggest problems dermatologists have in addressing the problem is that there is no medical textbook definition of "sensitive skin." This doesn't seem to deter cosmetic manufacturers from using the term freely, especially when they are trying to sell you so-called hypoallergenic cosmetics and other products for the skin that they claim are designed to deal with the condition.

Probably the most remarkable thing about the sensitive skin issue is that, for the most part, both the sufferer and the doctor don't really find much outwardly wrong with the skin. The bitter complaints of the sufferer appear far out of proportion to the medical findings. Precisely because so little is usually found, some doctors incorrectly label the whole condition psychosomatic. And as though that were not bad enough, the sufferer also eventually comes to believe that the whole problem is emotional.

Fortunately, ongoing research has begun to shed some new light on this condition. Based on their observations, some investigators have recently suggested that the sensitive skin problem be labeled the "status cosmeticus syndrome"; others prefer to call it "the intolerant skin syndrome." While these designations lend little to our understanding of the cause of the condition, they at least let the sufferer know that doctors are beginning to view the problem as something physiological rather than psychological.

Regardless of what it is called, however, the sensitive skin phenomenon seems to encompass a condition in which many, if not all, of the cosmetics that the sufferer applies to her face (the condition mostly affects women) produce some degree of tightness, burning, itching, or stinging, without any other objective (visible) findings. More severe cases may exhibit redness, irritation, mild swelling, and complexion changes, especially in the so-called butterfly area of the cheeks and eyelids. For some people, symptoms are limited to the eyes and usually consist of stinging and burning of the eyes and eyelids upon application of cosmetics in the eye area.

Diagnosing the sensitive skin or intolerant skin syndrome is further complicated by the fact that patch tests on the back with suspected allergy-provoking cosmetics and soaps are usually negative (nonreactive). Even "use" tests, in which small amounts of suspected culprits are repeatedly applied to the forearm for several days to look for possible reactions, also commonly prove negative. Rather than indicating that there is no organic problem, such a lack of reactivity may merely reflect the fact that facial skin microscopically differs from other skin areas, especially when it comes to irritant sensitivity to cosmetics. It is for this reason that doctors must maintain a very high index of suspicion for the sensitive skin condition in any person complaining of intolerance to lots of different kinds of topical products and cosmetics. At the same time, before they label the condition intolerant skin, they must make every effort to exclude the presence of subtle forms of eczema or other skin conditions that may be mimicking the problem.

Prevention

Given the difficulties in recognizing intolerant skin in the first place, it would seem fairly reasonable that treating the problem might prove equally daunting. In many instances it is a formidable challenge for both doctor and patient. Nevertheless, there are some broad commonsense recommendations that can be followed by those who are troubled with either sensitive skin or just sensitive eyelids.

Statistically, a number of common ingredients have been found to be particular troublemakers. If you believe you have intolerant skin, you would be wise to take great care in choosing products that contain them. Since researchers have determined that fragrances and sunscreen lotions together account for most cases of cosmetic-related itching, whenever possible you should look for fragrance-free products. It has also been determined that about 7 percent of the adult population experiences some form of adverse reaction to the common sunscreen ingredient PABA, and therefore you should select one of the PABA-free (and fragrance-free) sunscreens currently marketed (such as **Oil of Olay Daily UVA Protectant**).

You can also significantly reduce your need for sunscreens by rearranging your daily schedule and selecting proper outdoor attire to minimize sun exposure. For example, you might plan to stay out of the sun between the high-intensity hours of 10:00 A.M. to 3:00 P.M. and instead schedule your tennis or swimming before or after those times. You can also protect yourself by wearing special lightweight ultraviolet ray-shielding clothing (such as **Solumbra**, **Solar Protective Factory**, and **Frogskin**) that claims to yield protection equivalent to a sunscreen with an SPF of 30 or higher.

Other common ingredients capable of producing stinging and itching that are found in many different types of cosmetics should also be avoided if possible. These include benzoic acid, bronopol, cinnamic acid, Dowicil 200, formaldehyde, lactic acid, nonionic emulsifiers, propylene glycol, quaternary ammonium compounds, sodium lauryl sulfate, sorbic acid, and urea. A quick check of any product label will tell you if any of these are ingredients, and you can then look for alternatives.

If your problem is eyelid sensitivity, you may have a particularly difficult time finding a mascara that you can tolerate. Water-based mascaras that contain soaps and emulsifiers, such as sodium borate and ammonium stearate, can be especially problematic. If you have been having trouble with this kind, you might try a waterproof mascara. And if you still have problems, you may be able to use a cake mascara, although these are difficult to find nowadays.

Eye shadows, eyeliners, and artificial eyelashes can also cause problems for those with sensitive skin. Since they can be especially irritating, you should avoid frosted, pearlized, shiny, and glittery eye shadows, which usually contain fish scale fragments, bismuth oxychloride, mica, or ground metal particles. Look instead for those that give a matte or dull finish. And because their fluid bases tend to be less irritating, powdered eye shadows are preferable to the liquid or automatic pencil varieties. For the same reason, pencil and cake eyeliners are preferable to liquid ones. Lastly, the methacrylate-based (Krazy Glue-like) adhesives that are used to affix artificial lashes can aggravate sensitive eyelids and should be avoided entirely.

Interestingly, some researchers have suggested that the stinging effect of irritants in cosmetics may be countered by including so-called antiirritant ingredients in the products. At least in theory, antiirritants may work by combining directly with the irritants to neutralize them, blocking the specific sites where the irritants bind, or simply acting as physical barriers to prevent contact between the irritants and the skin. Antiirritants currently available include Polysorbate 20, aloe vera gel, Germall 115, imidazolidinyl urea, allantoin, and imidazolidine amphoteric surfactants (the cleansers used in the "no tears" shampoos). The jury is not yet in on the overall value of these agents as antiirritants.

If you complain of sensitivity on areas other than just your eyelids or face, you should be careful to choose gentle cleansers designed for use on the whole body (such as **Oil of Olay Sensitive Skin Bar**) and also hypoallergenic moisturizers for these areas. In addition, take quick showers, two to three minutes at most, to avoid overdrying and compounding the irritation problem. If you prefer baths to showers, add a little bath oil (such as **Alpha Keri**) to the water and do not use bubble bath products since they tend to be quite drying. And finally, use mild enzyme-free, dye-free, and perfume-free laundry detergents for your clothes, such as **Cheerfree** or **Ivory Snow**.

Treating Intolerant Skin

To reduce further irritation, eliminate washing your face with soaps or detergents. Instead, cleanse with only plain tepid water whenever possible. In general, you may continue to use lipstick and other lip cosmetics because they rarely cause problems for sensitive skin. You may also continue to use face powder since it, too, seldom aggravates the condition. If you are fortunate enough not to have a concurrent eyelid sensitivity, you may continue to use all your usual eyelid and eyebrow cosmetics.

If you need a moisturizer, you can experiment with the all-purpose kinds that are designated fragrance-free, such as **Curel** moisturizing lotion. Should even these prove irritating, you may have to resort to using plain glycerin and rose water, which can be purchased at most pharmacies. And lastly, a word of caution: Despite the extreme temptation, especially when you have some big social event coming up, you should refrain from using all other kinds of skin care cosmetics for at least six months or, better still, twelve months to allow your skin to fully recuperate. If you do this, your patience and forbearance may be rewarded by your being able to use your regular cosmetics once again on occasion without experiencing a recurrence of the skin problem.

CONTACT DERMATITIS

Since most information on adverse reactions to cosmetics is obtained from consumer complaints to the cosmetic manufacturer or to the FDA, the precise incidence of these problems is not really known. Many consumers who have a problem with one product or another simply switch brands in a trial-and-error fashion without letting anyone know. Considering the enormous number of people using so many different kinds of cosmetics during their lifetimes (millions of people use them every day), the actual total number of adverse reactions to cosmetics is believed to be surprisingly small. Of these, irritant rather than true allergic contact allergies make up the greatest proportion, more than 90 percent. This means that only about one in every ten reactions to cosmetics is a true allergic reaction. Occasionally, however, these reactions may be quite troublesome or severe, requiring medical attention.

Irritant Contact Dermatitis

Irritant contact reactions of the skin or nails, as opposed to allergic contact dermatitis, do not involve the immune system. Instead, as their name suggests, they are caused by direct irritation. For example, they may be provoked by such factors as excessive acidity or basicity (that is, too high or too low a pH) of a particular cosmetic or grooming agent. Highly alkaline toilet soaps, for example, especially if left in contact with the skin for too long a time, are well-known causes of direct irritation. Irritation is also far more likely to occur if potential irritants are applied to previously broken or diseased skin, and for this reason persons with excessively dry skin, atopic dermatitis, and psoriasis are particularly prone to such reactions.

Volatile substances that dissolve the protective oil layer of the skin and thereby expose it to greater irritation can also do it. Acetone and acetate, found in nail removers, and sodium or potassium hydroxide, which are ingredients in cuticle removers, are good examples of potential irritants that work in this fashion.

Mechanical factors that damage the skin surface and disrupt its protective barrier also predispose the skin to irritant dermatitis. Problems can result from the rubbing that may be required to apply a cosmetic or from the use of cosmetics containing abrasive particles. You are more likely to see this when soaps and cleansers that contain apricot pits or other ground abrasives are used.

Unfortunately, irritant reactions to cosmetics can sometimes be difficult to distinguish from true allergic reactions. Both may appear as itchy, reddish patches on the involved skin accompanied by blistering. As a rule, however, irritant reactions tend to appear within only a few hours of contact, whereas typical allergic reactions require at least two days or more to develop following contact with the offending cosmetic.

Treatment, like prevention, is a fairly simple matter of immediately discontinuing contact with the culprit product(s). This usually results in complete clearing within a few days. Occasionally, when the inflammation is severe, your doctor may need to prescribe a mild topical corticosteroid cream such as hydrocortisone to hasten clearing.

Allergic Contact Dermatitis

More than 50 percent of all cases of true allergies to cosmetics have been linked to the use of skin and hair care products and grooming agents that are intended to be left on the skin. The face and the region immediately around the eyes are the sites most often involved. Moisturizers, makeup, and sunscreens comprise the bulk of these "leave-on" products, and the fragrances and preservatives in them are most often the allergenic substances responsible for the adverse reactions. In general, as in the case of direct irritation, application of any product to previously inflamed skin increases the likelihood of adverse allergic reactions.

Of the most frequently used cosmetic ingredients, fragrances are the most common cause of allergic cosmetic allergy. In fact, scented products that are applied to skin which has become irritated or inflamed for one reason or another is believed to be responsible for most instances of cosmetic allergies. Products that contain fragrance— moisturizers, makeup, deodorants and antiperspirants, sunscreens, and, of course, perfume—have all been found capable of provoking these reactions.

Unfortunately, it is often difficult for fragrance allergy sufferers and their doctors to identify the scents that are responsible for the contact allergies. This is because fragrance formulations are often complex mixtures of chemicals, and many of these combinations are jealously guarded as "trade secrets" by the cosmetic and pharmaceutical houses that produce them. Some of the better known fragrance allergens include cinnamic alcohol, musk ambrette, hydroxycitronellal, isoeugenol, eugenol, geraniol, cinnamic aldehyde, and coumarin.

Note: Don't be fooled by the term *unscented* when searching for products that do not contain fragrances. Unscented and fragrance-free do not necessarily mean the same thing. While fragrance-free indicates that scents have been eliminated from the formulation altogether, unscented usually means that one or more scents have actually been *added* to a product with an otherwise medicinal or industrial aroma to render the final formulation less offensive to smell. Thus, if you are found to be allergic to fragrances, you should avoid scented products altogether and stick with fragrance-free items only.

Preservatives—the special ingredients used to prevent bacterial contamination and increase product shelf life—are the second most common cause of cosmetic contact allergy. Quarternium 15, a formaldehyde-releasing agent found in many moisturizers and hair care items, is a particularly common culprit in this category, and more than half of the individuals with quarternium 15 allergy are also allergic to formaldelhyde, another commonly used preservative. (For unexplained reasons, African-Americans have been found to be especially susceptible to this form of allergy.) Imidazolidinyl urea is the next most common cosmetic preservative allergen, followed by the parabens, 2-bromo-2-nitropropane-1, 3-diol, sorbic acid, diazolidinyl urea, MCI/MI (also listed on ingredient labels by its trade name, **Kathon CG**), glutaraldehyde, MGP (also known as **Euxyl K-400**), benzalkonium chloride, thimerosal, p-chloro-m-cresol, chloroxylenol, benzyl alcohol, sorbic acid, cetyl and stearyl alcohol, chloroacetamide, butylated hydroxyanisole (BHA), butylated hydroxytoluene (BHT), ethylenediaminetetraacetic acid (EDTA), and captan.

Lanolin (wool wax) and lanolin derivatives found in many commercial moisturizers and emollients make up another fairly large category of cosmetic allergens. In one study approximately 5 percent of all allergic reactions to cosmetics were related to these ingredients.

And lastly, the cosmetic allergens most often responsible for nail allergies include toluenesulfonamide/formaldehyde resin within nail enamels, free formaldelhyde in nail hardeners, methacrylate resins in sculptured and bonded nails, and the cyanoacrylate glues in nail repair kits.

Diagnosis

Contact rashes are typically red, scaly, itchy, and blistering. Although linking the outbreak of a rash to the use of a new cosmetic can be a simple matter when only a few cosmetics have been used, it may become difficult if you routinely use a wide variety of different cosmetics.

Finding the culprit can be even more difficult for your dermatologist when the allergic rash appears far from the actual site of application of the cosmetic. For example, you may be surprised to learn that nail polishes are responsible for many instances of allergic reactions around the eyes and eyelids (because the allergens are transferred there by your fingers). Similarly, nail polish may also be the cause of allergies on the legs if you use it to repair stocking runs. (Of course, allergies occur occasionally around the nails as well.) And allergies to shampoos or hair sprays typically show up as rashes on the neck, upper back, or forehead rather than the scalp, which is actually seldom affected by them. Considering the foregoing, a keen attention to detail is frequently required in order to make the correct diagnosis and isolate the real troublemaker(s).

When one or two cosmetics have been singled out as possible troublemakers, your doctor may suggest patch testing—placing a small amount of the suspected cosmetic on a patch and applying it to the skin of the inner upper arm or back to see whether the allergic rash is reproduced. If there is a reaction, your doctor may then contact the particular cosmetic manufacturer to obtain test amounts of the individual ingredients in the cosmetic for further patch testing. In this way the exact ingredient(s) that causes your allergy problem can be determined, and you can avoid purchasing all products that contain it in the future.

On the other hand, when a cosmetic allergy is suspected but no particular cosmetic can be singled out for blame, your doctor may recommend patch-testing you to all your cosmetics or to a standard screening tray that is composed of some of the more common allergens found in most cosmetics (see Appendix B).

Regardless of which method is used, once the allergy-provoking ingredients are determined, your doctor can provide you with a list of products that ordinarily contain them and advise you as to what alternatives (if any) exist and what other ingredients must also be avoided because they are chemically related to the ingredients to which you have been found allergic.

Prevention

Preventing allergic contact rashes is simple and can be summed up in one word: avoidance. In other words, you must do everything to limit further exposure. This is all the more important because inadvertent reexposure may trigger a more intense reaction and symptoms than the previous episode.

Sometimes you are able to get around your problem by simply switching to another cosmetic in the same category. For example, let's say you find yourself allergic to a particular brand of red blusher. First, you must stop using the blusher immediately and wait for the rash to clear completely. Next, you should choose another brand of red blusher and use it for three straight days. If you do not develop any problems, it is likely that you were allergic to some other ingredient in the blusher and not the pigment itself. You can then continue using the new product.

On the other hand, should you develop problems with the new red blusher, the red pigment may in fact be the culprit. In that case, once again let the allergy clear completely and then switch to a different color. If you do not develop any problems, the color was probably the allergen, and you must avoid that particular color blusher thereafter.

Should you once again develop allergic symptoms, however, the problem is most likely one or more of the many other ingredients that go into the cosmetic's manufacture. These include solvents, emollients, emulsifying agents (surfactants), preservatives, emulsion stabilizers, thickening and stiffening agents, chemical stabilizers, and antioxidants. And despite manufacturers' claims to the contrary, cosmetic formulations in the same category (that is, all blushers or all foundations) often share many of the same basic ingredients, which means that simply switching to another facial foundation may not solve your problem and may make trial-and-error testing a long, expensive, and frustrating ordeal. When this happens, you would be advised to consult a dermatologist about patch testing to specific ingredients, as described above.

Treatment

Topical corticosteroids are the mainstays of treating contact allergic rashes due to makeup, as they are for treating contact rashes due to other causes such as poison ivy. Usually only a short course of medium-potency products (for example, **Aclovate**, **Elocon**, **Locoid**, or **Westcort** creams) or low-potency products (for example, **Hytone 2.5%**) may be needed for between one and three weeks. High-potency steroids, because of their tendency to prematurely thin skin, are generally avoided on the more delicate skin of the face, especially the eyelids. Severe exudative and blistering rashes may additionally require a brief, tapering course of oral corticosteroids.

HYPOALLERGENIC COSMETICS

Although the term hypoallergenic when applied to any type of cosmetic may give the impression that the product is nonallergenic or at least much less allergenic than its competitors, this is not necessarily so. The origin of the term goes back about fifty years when a few companies began manufacturing cosmetics that did not contain ingredients that were commonly considered allergenic, such as certain fragrances. They called these cosmetics "hypoallergenic." Since that time, however, most manufacturers, particularly those in the United States, have realized that it makes good business sense to eliminate potential sensitizers from their products. After all, they are looking to hold on to their clientele as well. My favorite response when asked about hypoallergenic products versus their unlabeled counterparts is to ask, "Which manufacturer would produce products that were potentially highly allergenic to many people?" What can be said is that, to their credit, manufacturers of hypoallergenic product lines generally make their ingredient lists more readily available to physicians who request them. It bears repeating that regardless of whether a product carries the label hypoallergenic or not, there is no product yet available that is nonallergenic.

There is much to be said, however, for reducing the number of ingredients in any topical preparation, cosmetic, or medication. The more ingredients a product contains, the more potential there is for allergic sensitization. For that reason, be wary of products labeled herbal, natural, or organic. While the association with the freshness of Mother Nature is appealing, such products usually contain a host of unnecessary substances that add little to the overall benefit of the product but much to its potential for allergenicity.

Finally, don't be fooled by phrases such as *doctor-tested, dermatolo-*

gist-tested, or *allergy-tested*, which are so frequently used in cosmetic advertising. These nebulous terms are intended to snare you into a sense of security, but what they don't tell you is who did the testing, how the tests were done, or how many tests were actually performed. Without this kind of important information, you really have little assurance of the product's value or its true potential for irritancy or allergenicity.

CHAPTER TEN

GOING BUGGY: INSECT AND OTHER CRITTER ALLERGIES

For most people, flying and crawling insects and other bugs are a nuisance. They can ruin picnics, barbecues, and camping trips, and can make outdoor patio life downright miserable. But for others they are more than just "pesky critters," they are the source of all kinds of toxic and allergic problems and can even be lethal.

Bugs are well adapted to their roles and have evolved a variety of ways to cause us problems. Some sting us, injecting venom into our skin and bloodstream; others bite us, introducing saliva and other foreign materials; still others burrow and tunnel into and through the skin, depositing body proteins and waste materials capable of triggering all kinds of irritant and allergic reactions and infection. Some—most commonly house dust mites, crickets, and cockroaches—are capable of provoking severe allergic reactions and asthma attacks when their body parts or feces are inhaled by susceptible individuals. Naturally, location also plays an important role in determining what kinds of bug allergies are encountered most often. One might expect, for example, that city dwellers would be more likely to suffer cockroach allergies while rural populations would more likely suffer from bee stings.

While we often call every tiny winged or crawling creature an insect, technically insects are six-legged animals. Eight-legged animals, such as spiders and its relatives, are correctly called arachnids. Taken together, insects and arachnids are known as arthropods. All the varied kinds of reactions to bites and stings from arthropods as well as other animals could fill a book in itself, but the following will focus on some of the more common kinds of bug-related allergies.

THE BEE FAMILY

Although only about forty deaths from stinging insect reactions are reported every year, the figure is probably far higher. Also, perhaps surprisingly, it is double that of the number of deaths caused by poisonous snakes. Moreover, it is estimated that for every death that is reported there are thousands of severe and near-fatal reactions. The majority of these are caused by stings from a variety of common, mostly flying insects that belong to the order that scientists call the *Hymenoptera*. This large group includes yellow jackets, honeybees, hornets, wasps, and bumblebees. And of this group, more people die each year from bee stings than from all other insect attacks combined. Besides having membranous wings, all *Hymenoptera* possess venom-producing glands, located at the tip of the abdomen, through which they sting their victims to introduce the venom.

The *Hymenoptera* family also includes the ferocious imported fire ants that are found mostly in the southern United States; their sting, as the name suggests, feels like a sharp flash of fire. Distinct from its airborne relatives, however, these crawling insects (they do not fly despite the presence of wings) first bite their victims to lock on to them and then pivot their bodies to savagely deliver multiple stings.

As a rule, *Hymenoptera* sting only when frightened, although the so-called African killer bees, which have recently been migrating steadily upward from Mexico into the southern United States, are responsible for unprovoked attacks. Contrary to a popular misconception and despite what the name implies, the venom of killer bees is no more dangerous than that of its less aggressive relatives. Mild reactions to *Hymenoptera* stings, which consist of redness, slight swelling, tenderness, and mild pain at the sting sites, are not believed to be allergic in nature. Such reactions generally last no more than a few hours before subsiding completely without the development of any complications.

On the other hand, more extensive local reactions, such as those progressing to involve an entire arm or leg, as well as severe systemic reactions are felt to be allergy related. Two venom enzymes, *phospholipase* A and *hyaluronidase*, are believed to be the major allergens responsible for most allergic reactions to the bee family. It is also important to know that an allergy to one member of the *Hymenoptera* family may result in cross-allergies to other members of the group, and therefore if you have become sensitized to the yellow jacket, you may also develop a severe reaction to a wasp sting. Atopic individuals— those with a personal or family history of asthma, hay fever, or eczema—are more likely to develop true insect sting allergies than nonatopic persons. Severe swelling may be accompanied by intense itching, nausea, vomiting, abdominal cramps, dizziness, and wheezing. In extreme cases victims may suffer shock, a precipitous drop in blood pressure, and complete respiratory failure. These events often occur within thirty minutes of the sting. Because children tend to be less severely affected by systemic insect stings, most fatal reactions occur in adults.

Commonsense outdoor measures for protecting against stings include not wearing brightly colored clothing, flowery prints, or shiny jewelry; avoiding scented lotions, colognes, and hair sprays; and avoiding sweets, syrupy drinks, fruit juices, and sodas. In general, *Hymenoptera* are less attracted to white, green, and khaki colors. Obviously, wear your shoes and socks at all times, and never touch, sit, or step on anything outdoors without first looking. Commercial insect repellents are of little value against *Hymenoptera* and should not be relied on.

The best treatment for local reactions is rather simple: Remove the stinger and reduce the swelling. You can often get the stinger out by simply catching one of the barbs and scraping it out with the edge of a credit card or with your fingernail. This is particularly important if the sting is from a honeybee, which typically leaves its stinger behind. Don't use tweezers, and avoid any squeezing motions that might push more venom into the sting site.

Once you have removed the stinger, immediately elevate the affected area and apply ice. Additionally, if possible, within the first few minutes apply a small paste consisting of a few droplets of water and a commercial meat tenderizer. The protein-attacking enzyme *papain*, contained in the meat tenderizer, may help to reduce the swelling and pain, but only if it is used very soon after the sting. In uncomplicated cases swelling usually goes down in a day or so.

If the reaction is more severe and persistent, however, see your doctor. You may need a prescription for a topical corticosteroid cream and perhaps even an oral antihistamine such as chlorpheniramine (**Chlor-Trimeton**) or diphenhydramine (**Benadryl**) to reduce the inflammation and ease the symptoms. Acetaminophen (such as **Tylenol**) or ibuprofen (**Advil**) may also be helpful for reducing symptoms.

Severe allergic reactions require emergency care, which generally consists of the immediate injection of epinephrine (**Adrenalin**) and sometimes even the use of blood-pressure-elevating medications and respiratory assistance. Because of the tendency for symptoms to progress rapidly in these instances, time is of the essence. As a result, antihistamines and corticosteroid pills are of little value for emergency care since they begin working more slowly.

If you have a history of severe reactions to any *Hymenoptera* stings, you would do well to be evaluated by an allergist. Intradermal testing and RAST blood tests may be used to determine specific allergies to venom or venom components, although of the two methods, skin testing is more sensitive. Whatever method is selected, however, testing is usually postponed until at least six weeks after the last sting attack. This is to allow IgE antibody levels, which are depleted for several weeks following an attack, to return to normal.

Immunotherapy or desensitization shots (similar to the kinds used to treat hay fever allergies) have been shown to impressively reduce the risk of potentially life-threatening reactions to *Hymenoptera* stings—from 60 percent to as low as 5 percent. Desensitization is generally achieved by using specific venom proteins, the major allergenic culprits in most *Hymenoptera* problems. In the case of fire ants, however, since both the venom and the body proteins have been found to be allergenic, desensitization requires the use of whole body extracts of the bug.

In general, immunotherapy is reserved only for those who have a definite history of a systemic reaction to *Hymenoptera*. Because of the possibility of cross-allergenicity, many doctors choose to desensitize their patients with mixed-venom extracts. Shots are usually given about twice weekly for three months, and booster shots are generally given thereafter for the next five years to maintain adequate levels of immunity. A more rapid immunotherapy regimen is sometimes chosen, consisting of an entire series of increasing doses of venom administered over a several-hour period and followed by a series of four booster shots at periodic intervals. Many authorities recommend that maintenance venom immunotherapy be continued indefinitely.

Regardless of the precise method of desensitization, because protection is not absolute it is still advisable for anyone at risk of a life-threatening reaction to carry an emergency kit at all times outdoors (for example, **EpiPen**, **Ana-Guard**, or **Ana-Kit**). These kits usually contain antihistamine tablets, a tourniquet, a syringe, and most important, epinephrine ampules for self-injection. Careful attention should be paid to the package expiration date in order to replace the kit as needed. And since epinephrine may be affected by sunlight, the kit should be stored away from direct exposure. The user should of course be thoroughly familiar with the contents and their uses before heading out for a barbecue, picnic, or jaunt in the woods.

THE MOSQUITO FAMILY

Mosquitoes, biting flies, and gnats are all related, and much of what can be said about mosquitoes applies to the other two. Insects in this group cause injury by biting their victims rather than stinging them.

Accordingly, they provoke mechanical, toxic, and allergic reactions within the skin to the presence of their mouth parts and saliva. The actual severity of a person's reaction to mosquitoes and its relatives depends on how sensitive the person naturally is to them and how many times the person has been bitten before.

Mosquito bites are so common that almost everyone is familiar with their typical appearance. In most cases, shortly after the bite, a small, pale, pinkish hive appears, and it usually becomes redder and thicker within twenty-four hours before spontaneously disappearing. In sensitized persons, however, blisters may develop, and itching may become severe. Sometimes the sites of the bites grow into deep-seated nodules that eventually break down to form ulcerations in the skin and open the way for infection. Fortunately, systemic reactions rarely occur.

Prevention of bites from this group of insects follows many of the same commonsense rules discussed above for avoiding *Hymenoptera* attacks. Here again, you are advised to wear drab clothing and avoid scented products, including scented moisturizers and sunscreens. Leggings and veils, and the use of mosquito netting where appropriate, can also be helpful. More practically, DEET-containing insect repellents such as **Cutter** and **Off** have been shown to be quite effective, and they may be used safely on children. Serving a dual purpose, a relatively new product has come on the scene: **Vaseline Intensive Care's No Burn/No Bite**. An SPF 15, PABA-free sunscreen, this non-DEET product also contains a variety of ingredients that coat the skin and prevent mosquitoes from being attracted. It makes an ideal item to bring when picnicking, hiking, barbecuing, or camping, where both sun and bug protection are needed.

SCABIES

Scabies is a disease, or an infestation, caused by a nearly invisible creature: *Sacoptei scabiei*, better known as the "itch mite." The mite prefers to attack the thin-skinned regions of the body, those that are relatively free of hair and oil glands. Individuals of all ages and races are potential targets, and at present scabies is epidemic in the United States. Since it is spread through intimate body contact, scabies is currently one of the more prevalent sexually transmitted diseases and is especially common in persons under thirty.

The female itch mite, which burrows her home within her victim's skin, is the source of the problem. Linear zigzag burrows in which the female lays her eggs may range is size from one-eighth of an inch to several inches in length. As the organisms multiply and spread through the skin, small, pimplelike spots and tiny blisters or pustules begin to appear. Later, following an incubation period of about four to six weeks, a widespread rash covering large parts of the body may appear; it is intensely itchy, particularly at night. Scratch marks, crusting, and even infection may complicate the appearance of the rash. The eruption, which is believed to be allergic in nature, can be especially severe in individuals with a background of atopic dermatitis. (A less common variant, known as *nodular scabies*, in which thick, brownish red nodules form in the armpits, groin, buttocks, genital region, and shoulders, is also believed to have an allergic basis.)

Scabies is a highly contagious condition and usually spreads from one individual to another by direct contact. Even a simple handshake has been known to transfer the mite. It can also be spread through the sharing of clothing, particularly intimate apparel, towels, sheets, and pillow cases.

To diagnose scabies, a physician may scrape possible burrows and examine their contents under the microscope. Discovering adult mites or their eggs confirms a suspected case. Sometimes a physician will coat suspected burrows with a liquid tetracycline derivative and then examine the area with a special fluorescent light, known as a Wood's light, looking for the characteristic fluorescent yellow streak of a true burrow. A doctor rarely needs to biopsy a suspected site—that is, inject a small amount of local anesthetic to numb the area and then surgically remove a small piece of skin tissue to be examined under the microscope.

Fortunately, scabies can be cured quite easily these days. A relatively new topical medication, **Elimite**, a permethrin-containing compound, has proved safe and effective in eradicating most cases of the infestation and is today the treatment of choice. Lindane lotion (**Kwell**) and crotamiton lotion (**Eurax**) are effective alternatives. Regardless of the agent chosen, in order to be optimally effective it must be left on overnight. In addition to the medication, all bedclothes, sheets, towels, and linens must be dry-cleaned or laundered in hot water the morning after application in order to ensure destruction of all mites and to prevent reinfestation. Because of the high likelihood of spreading the infestation, other close family members should be examined and treated simultaneously to prevent a cycle known as "Ping-Pong" reinfestations. Finally, since itching often persists for days or even weeks after adequate treatment and destruction of the mites, you may have to continue oral antihistamines, topical anti-itch medications, and topical steroid creams during this period.

FLEAS

Fleas, one of man's peskiest attackers, are bloodsucking parasites that feed on dogs, cats, man, and many other animals. Unfortunately, we humans are susceptible to assault by fleas from other humans as well as by fleas from dogs and cats. Like body lice, fleas spend most of their time away from the host animal, attacking only periodically to feed. Flea saliva can be highly allergenic for some individuals.

Flea bites typically occur in groups or clusters on the arms, forearms, waist, buttocks, thighs, and lower legs. The ankles are an especially favored site. Individual bites appear pimplelike or hivelike and possess pinpoint-sized blood centers. Itching can be nerve-racking. In general, the severity of the skin reaction is a poor indicator of the number of fleas present. In other words, some people in contact with only a few fleas will develop severe allergic reactions, while others exposed to a heavy infestation may be completely symptom-free.

Topical corticosteroid preparations usually suffice to alleviate itching. On occasion oral antihistamines may be needed. But the trouble is far from over unless the fleas are eradicated. This is often no small task because fleas can remain alive for several weeks to as long as a year without feeding, and for every one seen on the body, there are probably between ten and one hundred others somewhere in the environment. This means that carpets, furniture stuffing, bedding, baseboards, and crevices where fleas typically reside need to be thoroughly sprayed with pyrethrin (**RID**) or commercial insecticides. Following that, you must vigorously vacuum these areas to remove surviving eggs and cocoons, which tend to be more resistant than adult fleas to the insecticides. Severe infestations of the home often require professional exterminators. Infested pets should of course be examined by a veterinarian and treated accordingly. Flea collars are not useful once your home has become infested and thus should not be relied on.

BEDBUGS

The common bedbug is a one-eighth-inch-long, six-legged, reddish brown creature. Like the mosquito, it feeds on blood by painlessly injecting a needlelike mouthpart into its victim's skin. It is typically a nighttime feeder, catching its victims asleep in bed (hence its name) and sensing its prey by either body heat or odor. Allergies to this bug are believed related to the bug's saliva, which it injects into the wound site to liquefy the skin and keep the blood from clotting.

Only one or two bite sites are typically found at a time. The face, arms, and legs—the exposed areas—are the favored sites of attack. The skin lesions that result are usually itchy round or oval hives that possess a small pinpoint-sized blood spot in the center. Especially susceptible persons may also develop small blisters and areas of eczema. More severe allergic symptoms include the development of widespread hives, asthma, and joint pains.

Bedbugs live in cracks and crevices within furniture and within any dark, insulated home area where they can hide. Like fleas, they can survive as long as one year without feeding. Bedbug infestations may be detected by the peculiar pungent odor in heavily infested dwellings or by identifying bedbug excrement on surfaces such as wallpaper.

As with other kinds of bites and sting reactions, local treatment usually consists of topical corticosteroid creams and oral antihistamines. More widespread reactions may also require oral corticosteroid pills such as prednisone to suppress inflammation. However, to put an end to the problem entirely rather than just treat symptoms, the bug must be rooted out of the home. Malathion- or pyrethrum-containing insecticides have proven effective for this. Unfortunately, because of this bug's incredible ability to hide and its mobility, extermination is often difficult even for professionals.

PAPULAR URTICARIA

Papular urticaria is a special form of hives that has been linked to the bites of a variety of insects and arachnids, including mosquitoes, fleas, and bedbugs. Not surprisingly, the problem is seasonal, generally occurring during the spring and summer, at the height of the bug season. It usually affects children between the ages of two and seven.

The eruption is marked by the appearance of waves of hivelike pimples ranging from one-eighth to one-half inch in diameter. The entire body may be affected, although most frequently lesions develop on the exposed areas of the face, neck, chest, backs of thighs, and buttocks. While some of the hives are found to possess a central prick mark, the site of an actual bite, the majority do not. The widespread nature of the eruption is believed to be an allergic reaction to only a few bites and is not the result of numerous bites all over.

In general, individual hives persist for between two to ten days, although occasionally the rash may persist for many weeks, even extending well beyond the end of the bug season. Recurrences are not uncommon, particularly in children with a personal or family history of atopy (asthma, seasonal rhinitis, or eczema).

The presence of seasonal, widespread, small-sized hives; a history of an exaggerated sensitivity to bug bites; and a personal or family history of atopy help to establish the diagnosis of papular urticaria. Preventive measures involve the same commonsense guidelines for avoiding biting and stinging insects described above. Treatment usually consists of the use of topical corticosteroid creams or lotions and oral antihistamines and corticosteroids.

HOUSE DUST BUGS

House dust is a complex mixture of, among other things lint, dander, fibers, mites, mite-derived feces, and insect parts. Overwhelming evidence points to the house dust mite, *Dermatophagoides* (literally, the skin eaters, because they feed on human skin dander), as the principal allergy-provoking element of house dust. These arachnids encase their feces in an intestinal enzyme-coated material that is thought to be the primary allergen for provoking the symptoms of perennial rhinitis and asthma.

Since mite fecal balls are relatively large and heavy, they float only very briefly in the air and settle quickly within "dust traps" such as carpets, bedding, and upholstery. Disturbing these sites, as for example during vacuuming, may result in a thirty-minute period of markedly increased airborne allergens and the possibility of eliciting inhalation allergy in sensitive individuals. Prevention and treatment therefore consist of dust-proofing the home environment as much as possible. This means eliminating carpets and other sites where mites thrive, emptying closets, encasing bedding, and frequently laundering curtains and bedding with hot water.

Cockroaches, the endemic pests of the urban dweller, are another major source of inhalation allergies. When these insects die naturally or are exterminated, their bodies slowly turn to a powdery material that becomes airborne. In addition, just as in the case of house mite feces, cockroach feces can also provoke allergy symptoms. Allergies to cockroaches should be considered in any urban dweller who suffers symptoms of perennial allergic rhinitis or asthma.

In theory, prevention and treatment of the problem is simple:

Eliminate the source. Unfortunately, cockroaches are extremely hardy organisms. For example, we know that one cockroach can survive on a tiny drop of water for a whole year. To date the only consistently effective measure for reducing exposure is periodic commercial extermination.

CHAPTER ELEVEN

IT CAN BE MURDER OUT THERE: ENVIRONMENTAL ALLERGIES

Like it or not, the technological world in which we live is filled with all kinds of poisons. It is a fact of modern industrial life and all too often a cause of death. Almost everywhere we turn we run into large and small factories belching out tons of smoke and debris into the air, adding to the tons continuously pouring out from the exhaust pipes of all our cars and jet aircraft. Add to this aerosol spray fumes and cigarette smoke, and we are talking about more than 150 million tons of air-polluting wastes spewed out each year over the United States and Canada alone.

Air pollution is not our only environmental enemy, however. While most of us have heard about the relationship between long-term sun exposure and the subsequent development of skin cancers and premature skin aging, few are aware that for some individuals the sun's ultraviolet rays can also trigger a wide array of allergic symptoms, either alone or when combined with the ingestion or application of certain substances or medications.

AIR POLLUTION AND ALLERGY SYMPTOMS

Air pollutants are a complex mixture of gases, including ozone, sulfur dioxide, nitrogen dioxide, carbon monoxide, and hydrocarbons. From one place to another the ratio of these compounds can vary significantly, depending on such factors as the kinds and numbers of automobiles in a given location, the number of smokers, the types of nearby factories, and the vagaries of the weather. For example, when warm air masses move over cooler surface air, a condition of stagnant, sometimes life-threatening pollution is created at low altitudes. This situation is particularly dangerous for persons with prior heart or respiratory problems.

Much remains to be learned about the mechanisms by which pollution harms us, but it is believed do so in one or more of several ways. It may be directly toxic to tissues, it may trigger the onset of new allergies, or it may aggravate preexisting ones. Researchers have accumulated convincing evidence that pollution can trigger or aggravate asthma as well as chronic bronchitis. Likewise, the irritating chemicals contained in hair sprays, air fresheners, and cleaning preparations have been found to make the symptoms of preexisting allergic nasal congestion and wheezing flare up in susceptible individuals. An allergic basis has been suggested to explain at least some of the cases of headache, weakness, and nausea that have been associated with the inhalation of gasoline and other hydrocarbon fumes. Since pollutants have been shown to be capable of triggering the release of histamine, the chemical mediator involved in many forms of allergic (as well as nonallergic) inflammatory reactions, some experts have suggested this as a possible explanation for some of these findings.

There is only one way to alleviate the problems related to air pollution: strict enforcement of Environmental Protection Agency (EPA) measures to reduce pollution, and automobile and factory emissions. Allergy-prone individuals and those with other respiratory problems are advised to stay indoors on high-pollution days and to rely on air-conditioning units whenever possible.

MULTIPLE CHEMICAL SENSITIVITY

As though contending with air pollution were not enough, there are individuals who suffer from what is called multiple chemical sensitivity (MCS). Most experts in environmental and occupational medicine restrict the diagnosis of this controversial condition to those who have developed an apparent supersensitivity to common environmental agents that cannot otherwise be readily explained by conventional medical or psychological diagnoses. Sometimes referred to as "environmental disease" or the twentieth-century syndrome, MCS is believed to be far from rare. The total number of sufferers in the United States is not known, but one recent study of patients visiting the occupational medicine clinics at two major medical centers suggested that the number of victims may be as high as 1 percent. While both sexes and any age group may be affected, the typical MCS sufferer is a white, middle-aged, middle- to upper-class woman.

Signs and symptoms of MCS include fatigue, dizziness, headache, memory loss, difficulty in concentrating, and mood alterations. Sufferers may also complain of rapid heartbeat, breathing difficulties, chest tightness, abdominal cramping, bloating, and diarrhea. Inflammation of the mucous membranes of the eyes, nose, and throat may also develop. Because the manifestations of MCS typically mimic those resulting from many other medical and emotional conditions, the diagnosis is often difficult to establish conclusively.

The list of substances that have been linked to MCS is awesome, and a detailed discussion of them would require a large volume in itself. The following are but a few of the more common categories of agents that have been implicated: *Aliphatic hydrocarbons,* found in glues and adhesives; *aromatic hydrocarbons,* which are in solvents and thinners such as benzene and toluene; *halogenated hydrocarbons,* contained in dyes, drugs, and disinfectants; *chlorines,* in bleaches and products in which bleaches are used, such as facial and toilet tissues, disposable diapers, tampons, and so forth; *Phenols,* found in preservatives, aerosol disinfectants, and oral hygiene products; *formaldehyde,* encountered in glues and resins, preservatives, chemical stabilizers, and permanent press and fireproof fabrics.

Persons affected by MCS are generally in good health until exposure to the particular environmental agent or type of environment that initiates the problem. At first the symptoms typically relate to the agent causing the problem. For example, the sensitive individual exposed to formaldehyde might complain of breathing difficulties and/or irritation of the eyes and skin. If exposure continues, lower concentrations of formaldehyde will trigger the same symptoms. Persistent exposure may ultimately give rise to what has been termed the "spreading phenomenon" in which the same symptoms once exclusively linked to the formaldehyde are now provoked by an ever-growing list of other substances or types of environments. These can include the scents of perfumes, cigarette smoke, new upholstery, carpets, pesticides, and news print, and may occur even in grocery store aisles or shopping malls. Curiously, this phenomenon can develop even when there has never been a problem with any of these items or places before. In general, MCS tends to be chronic, progressive, and severely debilitating. On rare occasions the condition has spontaneously disappeared as mysteriously as it appeared.

Experts disagree as to the underlying causes of MCS. Some theorize a hereditary basis. Others suggest that it is idiosyncratic in origin, that there is something peculiar to the makeup of the sufferer that is at fault. Still others contend that MCS is an allergic reaction. The latter maintain that the apparently nonspecific responses of victims to so many different environmental agents is in reality a consistent response to a single, as yet unidentified, ubiquitous allergen.

But whatever the precise cause(s) of MCS, diagnosing it is difficult. Unfortunately, no specific diagnostic laboratory tests are currently available. Allergists and specialists in both environmental medicine and occupational medicine generally agree on the following criteria for diagnosing MCS:

1. The symptoms must involve more than one organ system and must be aggravated by environmental agents or environments that do not affect the vast majority of the population.
2. The problem must have been present at least three months.
3. There must be no other medical or psychological conditions that would account for the patient's complaints.

In addition to a complete medical history and physical examination, a comprehensive workup for MCS might include allergy testing, dietary manipulation, pulmonary function studies, and smell acuity testing, depending on individual circumstances.

For the present, treatment of MCS basically consists of avoiding any known triggering factors and using medications to relieve symptoms. Suggested measures for improving the quality of the home environment are those recommended for dealing with traditional respiratory allergies and asthma (see chapters 2 and 5). Perhaps the most encouraging bit of news for sufferers is the apparent growing recognition of MCS in the United States as a real entity that deserves additional intense investigation.

SICK-BUILDING SYNDROME

Related to air pollution and perhaps to MCS, another environmental condition has come to be known as the "tight-building" or "sick-building" syndrome (SBS). Recognized since the 1970s, this condition is very much an outgrowth of our late-twentieth-century cost consciousness and emphasis on energy efficiency. The World Health Organization (WHO) defines sick-building syndrome as an excess of work-related irritations of the skin and mucous membranes and of a variety of other symptoms, especially headache, fatigue, and difficulty concentrating. SBS is associated with newly constructed or remodeled, tightly sealed, climate-controlled buildings, hence the name.

To improve energy efficiency, ventilation systems in newer or remodeled homes have been designed to pull in less fresh outdoor air and recirculate more indoor air. Although they are more energy and cost efficient, such systems result in elevations in the concentrations of indoor pollutants and other contaminants. Not surprisingly, SBS occurs more frequently in buildings where ventilation rates are set near the minimum, and for that reason the American Society of Heating, Refrigeration, and Air Conditioning Engineers has repeatedly recommended increases in the minimal supply of outdoor air per person per minute. The issue is far from settled or clearly understood, however, since data from a recent research investigation published in the prestigious *New England Journal of Medicine* did not demonstrate any improvement in the symptoms of sufferers when supplies of fresh air were increased.

Whatever the actual causes, the extent of the problem is not believed to be small. The WHO estimates that SBS occurs in as many as 30 percent of new and remodeled office buildings. This translates into a problem that may affect approximately one million modern commercial buildings in the United States. If this is indeed so, between 30 million and 70 million employees are potential victims.

Upper respiratory tract symptoms, including stuffy or runny noses, coughing, sneezing, sore throat, shortness of breath, and chest tightness are among some of the many symptoms of people complaining of SBS. Headache, excessive tiredness, sore eyes, itching, dry skin, and skin rash have also been ascribed to the syndrome. Curiously, women tend to be more affected than men, and nonsupervisory personnel more than management-level employees. Unlike the case with multiple chemical sensitivities, the manifestations of sick-building syndrome do not include food intolerances or gastrointestinal problems. Typically, all symptoms of SBS improve or disappear entirely whenever the sufferer is away from the building environment.

The precise agents responsible for SBS are not known. However, a closed environment allows for the proliferation of a wide variety of germs and for the concentration of allergens and other irritating airborne particles, all or a combination of which may be responsible. Examples of potential problem-causers include cigarette smoke, perfumes, pesticide fumes, molds, mites, carbonless paper, fabric particles, and fiberglass, to name just a few.

As in the case of multiple chemical sensitivities, diagnosing sick-building syndrome and finding its particular causes can be difficult. While no specific, objective diagnostic laboratory tests are available, samples of air may be taken to determine levels of carbon dioxide, the major component of exhaled air. If nothing else, an elevated level would suggest inadequate ventilation. Finding clusters of individuals who are suffering with symptoms of the syndrome rather than isolated cases is another strong supportive piece of evidence that something may be amiss in their common environment.

It goes without saying that better designed and maintained ventilation systems are needed to improve the internal environments of many of our modern office buildings. Closer attention to the choice of construction materials as well as to the products we use in the workplace (just as in the home) can also go far in reducing the levels of potential toxins and allergens.

HYPERSENSITIVITY PNEUMONITIS

Hypersensitivity pneumonitis is a fancy way of saying allergic lung inflammation. The condition is not really one illness but a group of illnesses that share the same constellation of signs and symptoms with differing specific allergic causes. Based on the particular route of allergen entry into the body, hypersensitivity pneumonitis has been called by a variety of other names, including farmer's lung, ventilation pneumonitis, bird breeder's lung, and chemical worker's lung. In general, whatever the cause, the condition develops after months to years of strong exposure to the allergen.

Depending on whether allergenic exposure is of short duration or persistent, hypersensitivity pneumonitis may follow either an acute or a chronic course. In the acute (short-duration) variety, symptoms typically arise within a few hours of exposure and generally consist of cough, shortness of breath, and flulike symptoms such as fever, chills, muscle aches, and extreme tiredness that last for only one or two days. Progressive shortness of breath and increasing physical disability, however, characterize the chronic (long-term) variety.

Farmer's lung has been linked to exposure to moldy hay, which contains contaminant bacteria believed to be directly responsible for provoking the allergic symptoms. In this condition the bacteria operate as allergens rather than as infective germs. In the same way ventilation pneumonitis is associated with bacterial and fungal contamination of the water in humidifiers and air conditioners. Here again the germs act as allergens rather than infection-producing agents. Bird breeder's lung is a potential hazard for those raising pigeons, parakeets, chickens, and turkeys. The problem is believed to result from breathing in the dried, powdery fecal material deposited by the birds. And in chemical worker's lung, the symptoms have been tied to inhalation of *isocyanates*, which are present in polyurethane foam, varnishes, and lacquers.

In most cases, hypersensitivity pneumonitis is a relatively mild illness. When exposure to the provocative allergen is short-lived, the chances for complete recovery are generally excellent. On the other hand, a history of repeated acute episodes presages a worse prognosis. The outcome is also poorer when the hypersensitivity pneumonitis is severe and long-term enough to cause persistently abnormal chest X-ray findings and lung function studies. Somewhat surprisingly, there is a tendency in chronic cases for the severity of symptoms to decrease over time.

The treatment of choice for hypersensitivity pneumonitis, as for most allergic disorders, is avoidance of the allergen. However, as many as 60 percent of farmers and an even greater percentage of bird breeders with the condition are financially unable to give up their work. At the very least these individuals must avoid baling or storing *wet* hay and should use filter masks or respirators whenever they are exposed. Two choices of filter masks include the disposable 3M model 8710 and the reusable model 7200. Storage driers to reduce moisture buildup and spraying with propionic acid are other effective methods of reducing the bacterial contamination responsible for the problem. Finally, short courses of antiinflammatory steroids such as prednisone may also be used to break the ongoing cycle.

Persons suffering with ventilation pneumonitis would do well to avoid standing water in air-conditioning and humidification units and to make certain that local reservoirs are properly treated to suppress bacterial overgrowth. Finally, chemical workers can reduce their overall exposure by not handling dusty materials within small, closed spaces and ensuring that all standards for proper ventilation are being adhered to in the workplace.

PHOTOALLERGIES

As though it weren't enough to worry about the air we breathe, both in and out of doors, some people must also worry about allergies to sunlight. A dermatologist once observed that one of the greatest mysteries is the development in an otherwise healthy person of an allergy to something as essential to life on earth as the sun's rays. Nevertheless, it does occur. In some instances a topically applied substance or an internal medication is responsible for making the individual more sunsensitive. But in other cases the sun's ultraviolet radiation alone is enough to trigger hives or other allergic reactions.

Scientists refer to all adverse reactions to the sun as *photosensitivity reactions*. Those reactions that are sunburnlike, whether they are caused directly by the ultraviolet rays or the combination of the radiation and some chemical applied to the skin or ingested, are known as *phototoxic reactions*. Ordinary sunburn is the most common example of a phototoxic reaction. Those that involve the immune system on an allergic basis are known as *photoallergic reactions*.

Photoallergies occur much less commonly than phototoxic reactions, although as a rule they require less radiation energy to trigger them. These reactions may be either of the immediate hypersensitivity kind or the delayed allergic kind (see Chapter 1). *Solar urticaria* and *polymorphous light eruption* are two photoallergic conditions that result from ultraviolet radiation alone. *Photoallergic contact dermatitis* and *systemic photoallergy*, on the other hand, result from the interaction of ultraviolet radiation and a topical or ingested chemical or medication.

Solar Urticaria

Solar urticaria is just a fancy way of referring to hives that are induced by exposure to the sun. Although not yet conclusively proven to be at fault, IgE antibodies are believed to be involved in at least some cases. The condition most commonly affects those between the ages of twenty and forty.

Sun-induced hive reactions typically occur within seconds to minutes following exposure and may last for minutes to hours, depending on the intensity of the ultraviolet radiation. Under the microscope and even to the naked eye, the hives produced by ultraviolet light are no different from those that are caused by foods or drugs. Although spontaneous remissions do occur, solar urticaria more frequently persists for life.

Diagnosing solar urticaria is usually a straightforward matter: The patient gives a history of breaking out in hives after being in the sun. To confirm the diagnosis, the dermatologist may perform *phototesting*. The simplest form of phototesting involves exposing a small area of the patient's skin for the amount of time the person claims causes his reaction. The development of hives following such exposure confirms the diagnosis.

Most people with solar urticaria are extremely sensitive to the sun, making treatment a challenge. Unquestionably, the preventive measures of avoidance of sun exposure and the use of protective clothing whenever outdoors are the best forms of treatment. Sunscreens have proven inadequate for most people with the condition, but the non-sedating antihistamine terfenadine (**Seldane**) has been shown to be helpful in certain cases.

Polymorphous Light Eruption

Polymorphous light eruption (PMLE) is another allergic condition related to ultraviolet light alone. It is the most common light-related eruption in North and Central America and Great Britain. The problem may arise at any time of life but most frequently begins sometime before the age of thirty.

The term "polymorphous," which literally means "many forms," refers specifically to the many kinds of skin problems that may be seen in persons with this condition. These include reddish, pimplelike bumps, blisters, eczemalike patches, and large, deep-seated nodules and plaques. In most instances the skin eruptions begin within twenty-four to forty-eight hours of sun exposure and persist for several days. The delayed time frame from exposure to skin rash suggests a delayed hypersensitivity mechanism (see Chapter 1).

As in the case of solar urticaria, the diagnosis rests heavily on a history of delayed reaction to sun exposure. Phototesting may be helpful in confirming suspected cases.

Fortunately, most people with PMLE have a mild form of the condition and require no therapy at all. Such people typically experience one or two episodes of the problem each year in the early spring and, for reasons that remain obscure, become resistant to the ill effects of the sun for the remainder of the spring and summer seasons. More difficult cases may respond to the use of topical and systemic corticosteroid agents such as prednisone. Certain antimalaria drugs have also proven quite effective. Most recently, the anticancer drug azathioprine (Imuran) was demonstrated to be valuable for treating middle-aged and older patients with the PMLE's eczema variant.

Photocontact Dermatitis

The essential difference between allergic contact dermatitis (as discussed in Chapter 7) and photoallergic contact dermatitis is that the latter requires ultraviolet A (UVA) radiation *in addition to* a light-sensitizing topical agent in order to provoke an allergic attack. Since UVA penetrates glass, a susceptible individual may be exposed while driving, while sitting indoors next to a window, and even while wearing a sunscreen that has inadequate UVA protectants. Some well-known photoallergens include certain colognes, aftershaves, and perfumes (that have, for example, musk ambrette, sandalwood oil, and 6-methyl coumarin); Persian lime rind; diphenhydramine (for example, **Benadryl** spray); epoxy resins; and halogenated salicylanalides (antibacterial and antifungal agents). Nowadays, ironically, sunscreens containing PABA, PABA esters, or oxybenzone are the leading causes of photocontact dermatitis. And since sunscreen ingredients are also commonly found in moisturizers and makeup, these products must be kept in mind when looking for potential sources of photocontact allergies.

In a small percentage of people with photoallergic contact dermatitis, the disease may progress to the point where they continue to develop photoallergic reactions to sunlight in the absence of further contact with the topical agent that originally triggered it. When this occurs, dermatologists refer to the condition as *persistent light reaction*.

Although protected areas of skin are occasionally involved, not surprisingly the sun-exposed areas of the body are the favored sites for photocontact allergy. Nonexposed areas, such as the upper eyelids, the skin behind the ears, and the neck folds, are typically spared. Adults are much more commonly affected than children. Possible allergic reactions include redness and severe blistering, although eczema is the most common manifestation.

While the typical history and clinical examination may suggest the diagnosis, photopatch testing establishes it. In this test duplicate amounts of the suspected topical photoallergens are applied to the skin. After twenty-four hours one set of allergens is irradiated with UVA, and at forty-eight and seventy-two hours the irradiated and nonirradiated sides are examined. Reproducing the allergic skin rash at the irradiated site confirms the diagnosis (see Appendix A).

Therapy for photocontact dermatitis is identical to that used in ordinary allergic contact dermatitis. The mainstays include oral antihistamines and topical and oral corticosteroids (see Chapter 7). Except in cases of persistent light reaction, avoidance of the photoallergen(s) will prevent recurrences. Sun protection measures are crucial for controlling persistent light reactions.

Systemic Drug Photoallergy

Although much less common than photoallergic contact dermatitis, allergic reactions resulting from the combination of ultraviolet light and a *systemic* medication (rather than a topical agent) do occur. A large number of agents has been associated with this type of allergy, including sulfonamides (antibiotics such as **Gantrisin, Septra,** and **Bactrim**); sulfonylureas (oral antidiabetic drugs such as **Tolinase** and **Orinase**); thiazide diuretics (such as **HydroDIURIL**); quinidine (a heart rhythm regulating drug such as **Quinaglute**); phenothiazines (such as **Thorazine**); oral contraceptives; griseofulvin (antifungal agents such as **Fulvicin** and **Gris-Peg**); several antihistamines; and piroxicam (**Feldene**). Reddish flat-topped bumps and eczema are the most common types of skin eruptions seen in this condition. In general, photoallergic systemic reactions are of the delayed allergy type and thus begin twenty-four to forty-eight hours after UV exposure.

The diagnosis of photoallergic drug reaction is usually made from the history and clinical picture. Occasionally, phototesting may also be helpful in confirming the diagnosis.

Prevention and treatment require either discontinuing the offending medication or avoiding sun exposure. Unfortunately, depending on the particular drug involved, in some cases it may take as long as three to four months for the drug to clear the body and for the symptoms to disappear completely. Of course, when a particular drug is essential for the treatment of a serious medical condition and no equivalent substitution is available, sun avoidance becomes the only alternative. Specific treatment measures are the same as those for photocontact allergy.

CHAPTER TWELVE

BEING ALLERGIC TO YOURSELF: AUTOIMMUNE DISORDERS

For most people the concept of being allergic to something, for example to a drug, food, or poison ivy, is not particularly hard to understand and accept. On the other hand, the idea of being allergic to yourself is a much more difficult notion to grasp. Nevertheless, a surprising number of allergies of this kind do occur. Immunologists call these reactions autoimmunity (literally, immunity against self), and allergic disorders of this variety are known collectively as autoimmune disorders.

The natural question arises: How can someone be allergic to himself or herself and still live? The fact is, many autoimmune disorders are serious and even life-threatening and require intensive medical therapy for lives to be saved. Immunologists and rheumatologists, the medical specialists most concerned with these diseases, would probably be the first to admit that while much progress has been made in diagnosis and treatment over the last quarter of a century, much more remains to be learned about autoimmune disorders.

Some of the growing list of diseases that have been associated with autoimmunity are as follows:

1. A wide variety of blistering diseases of the skin, including pemphigus and pemphigoid
2. Acute rheumatic fever, a special form of heart disease

3. Certain neurologic and muscular disorders, such as multiple sclerosis and myasthenia gravis

A detailed discussion of these and the many other conditions linked to self-allergy is well beyond the scope of this book, but in this chapter I hope to give you a broad overview of some of the more common conditions in this category. This includes a group of diseases known as collagen vascular disorders; two relatively common glandular conditions, Hashimoto's thyroiditis and juvenile-onset diabetes; and two well-known dermatologic conditions, vitiligo and alopecia areata.

COLLAGEN-VASCULAR DISORDERS (ARTHRITIC DISEASES)

This category of conditions comprises a variety of diseases in which autoimmunity was first suspected and the notion articulated. It is composed of *systemic lupus erythematosus* (often called "lupus" or SLE for short), *rheumatoid arthritis, progressive systemic sclerosis* ("scleroderma"), and *dermatomyositis*, among others. Although each of these conditions is a distinct disease, they are grouped together because they have similar signs and symptoms and, in certain cases, overlapping laboratory abnormalities. The common manifestation of arthritis in victims of these disorders accounts for the name of the specialty that most often deals with them: *rheumatology*, or the study of joint diseases.

Lupus

Lupus is considered the prototype autoimmune disease, and investigators maintain that understanding this condition better will lead to more effective ways to diagnose and treat other autoimmune conditions. It is a fairly common disorder, developing overall in about one in every two thousand people. The disease has a predilection for women, affecting approximately one in every seven hundred white women and one in every two hundred forty-five black women between the ages of twenty and sixty-five. The precise cause is unknown, although genetic factors are believed to play a role. Hormonal, stress, and viral factors may also help to trigger flare-ups or aggravate preexisting disease.

The signs and symptoms of lupus are diverse and reflect the fact that autoantibodies (that is, antibodies that attack the self) may be produced against many different tissue and organ components. One variant of lupus that involves only the skin, *discoid lupus erythematosus*, is typically a scarring, disfiguring condition. SLE, on the other hand, is characterized by much more widespread organ involvement. In addition to fever, fatigue, weight loss, and loss of appetite, SLE sufferers may experience facial and body rashes, heightened sun sensitivity, canker sore-like irritations in the mouth and nose, arthritis (joint inflammation, swelling, and pain), and kidney, lung, nerve, and blood system problems.

Diagnosing lupus requires a thorough history and physical examination combined with a sophisticated immunologic blood workup. The *antinuclear antibody* test, usually referred to as the ANA *titer*, is a highly sensitive screening test for lupus. The test derives its name from the fact that the antibodies are directed specifically at the material within the nucleus of the victim's own cells. To confirm the diagnosis additional tests are often needed.

Since no cure yet exists, treatment is directed at relieving symptoms and prolonging life. Systemic corticosteroids and premier antiinflammatory agents such as prednisone are the mainstays of therapy. Occasionally other antiinflammatory drugs, such as aspirin, indomethacin (**Indocin**), and antimalarial agents (such as chloroquine and hydroxychloroquine) may be prescribed. Happily, more than 90 percent of patients today survive more than fifteen years with that condition that at one time was almost universally fatal. For further information, write The National Lupus Erythematosus Foundation, 2635 North First Street, Suite 206, San Jose, California 95134.

Rheumatoid Arthritis

To the general public rheumatoid arthritis (RA) is probably the best known autoimmune disorder. Affecting three times as many women as men, it is a chronic, often relapsing disease that may involve any combination of joints. In advanced cases it is a deforming, often severely disabling and potentially life-threatening condition. As in the case of lupus, an inherited susceptibility is believed to be a factor in its development. The possible contributing roles of viral infection, stress, and hormonal factors remain to be elucidated. The initial autoallergic (autoimmunologic) site of attack involves the *synovium*, the membranelike tissue covering of the joints.

In most cases the symptoms of rheumatoid arthritis first appear between the ages of thirty-five and forty-five. Small, medium, or large joints, such as the fingers, wrists, elbows, knees, and hips, may be involved alone or in any combination. Joint involvement is often symmetrical, meaning that, for example, both knees or both wrists are usually involved simultaneously.

Early in the course of the disease, sufferers usually complain only of low-grade fever, fatigue, weight loss, glandular swelling, and morning stiffness in their joints. Thereafter, however, symptoms progress either slowly or rapidly. In long-standing cases, muscular contractures (severe stiffening and irreversible contractions of the muscles) may occur and lead to all kinds of characteristic skeletal deformities. Some of these deformities have been given descriptive names because of their striking physical appearance—for example, the "swan neck" or "cock-up toes" deformities of the hands and feet.

In addition to joint problems, patients with rheumatoid arthritis may suffer with inflammation of the outer lining tissues of the lungs and heart (*pleuritis* and *pericarditis*, respectively); nerve, eye, and blood vessel problems; and the development of skin nodules and ulcerations.

The diagnosis of rheumatoid arthritis requires a thorough history and physical examination, looking for the presence of at least several of the above manifestations. The *rheumatoid factor* test is the major blood-screening examination for this condition. A negative test (that is, one in which the rheumatoid factor is not found) does not exclude the diagnosis, however, since it may be absent in as many as 20 percent of those who fit the other criteria for rheumatoid arthritis. Nonetheless, it is an excellent screening examination. Questionable cases require the use of other, often more sophisticated immunologic blood testing. X-ray examination, looking for the destructive changes typical of RA, are also helpful.

The course of the disease is unpredictable. As many as 20 percent of patients are fortunate enough to experience a complete disappearance of the problem or only mild, occasional flare-ups of the condition. On the other hand, approximately 10 percent suffer progressive crippling. The vast majority of persons with the condition fall somewhere in between these two extremes.

For persons with mild to moderate disease, rest, physical therapy, and the use of high-dose aspirin or other nonsteroidal antiinflammatory agents (such as **Motrin**, **Naprosyn**, or **Indocin**) may be sufficient to control symptoms and improve the quality of life. For more resistant cases, occasional use of low doses of oral corticosteroids (prednisone) and the injection of corticosteroids directly into affected joints may provide dramatic relief for prolonged periods of time. A number of other potent systemic agents are available in the event that these measures prove inadequate. For advanced cases, treatment is challenging, and management requires an interdisciplinary approach that ideally involves a team of rheumatologists, dermatologists, physical therapists, occupational therapists, psychologists, and surgeons. For more information contact the Arthritis Foundation, 1314 Spring Street, N.W., Atlanta, Georgia 30309.

Scleroderma

Scleroderma, or progressive systemic sclerosis (PSS), is another fairly well-known autoimmune disorder, affecting nearly three-quarters of a million Americans. The term *sclerosis*, which means thickening of the skin, refers to the primary feature of this disease, the laying down of excessive amounts of fibrous tissue within the skin as well as other organs of the body. Abnormal changes in certain blood vessels throughout the body are another characteristic of the disorder. Scleroderma shows no racial preferences, but it does affect three times as many women as men. Symptoms most often appear first in the patient's twenties or thirties. Current evidence points to an autoimmune basis, although the specific triggering cause(s) are not yet known. Environmental exposures, such as exposure to polyvinyl chloride or to silica, may also play some role, at least in some cases.

The manifestations of scleroderma within the skin generally pass through three stages. The first stage is the development of stiffness and nonpainful swellings, which may be confined to the hands or may affect the entire body. In the second stage, the sclerotic or so-called hidebound stage, affected skin becomes extremely dry, taut, smooth, waxy, and leathery. The patient's face typically loses its wrinkles and folds, assuming an artificial masklike appearance. At the same time, the tautness of the skin over the fingers and other joints limits their full extension. In the final stage, paradoxically, the skin may become abnormally thin and may even soften somewhat. Scleroderma that affects only localized patches of skin without any other organ involvements is generally a much milder condition known as *morphea*, which has an excellent prognosis.

When it extends to other organs, the abnormal fibrosing process of scleroderma results in, among other things, inflamed muscles, joint contractures, abnormal movement in the esophagus (often creating swallowing problems), and a condition known as *Raynaud's phenomenon*, a dramatically increased sensitivity to cold. Preceding the onset of any other symptoms in more than 50 percent of all scleroderma patients, Raynaud's phenomenon results from spasms within the small blood vessels of the fingers and toes and manifests as an abnormal and prolonged sequence of turning white, red, and blue in response to being in a cold environment or when holding ice or even a cold drinking glass.

As mentioned earlier, patients with scleroderma typically develop thick hidebound skin above the wrists and tightly flexed fingers. When these are present, the diagnosis is usually not difficult. By contrast, accurately diagnosing a patient in the early stages when there is no skin involvement can be extremely difficult. A number of antibody blood tests are employed in the diagnosis of scleroderma. Although not an especially sensitive screening test, the *antinucleolar antibody* test, which looks for antibodies directed to the nucleolus, a special portion of the nucleus of the cell, is the most specific blood examination for scleroderma. In certain cases a variety of other antibody tests may also be ordered. Abnormalities in the pattern and distribution of the tiny blood vessels in the nail folds of the fingers is another good indication of scleroderma, and these may even be present before the development of the full-blown disease. Finally, where appropriate, doctors may order special X-ray and pressure studies (manometric tests) of the esophagus to search for abnormal motility (movement) problems.

Although episodic spontaneous improvement does occur, scleroderma generally follows a relentless, chronic course. Those patients with mainly skin involvement tend to have a slower progression of their disease than others in whom the disease involves the kidneys, lungs, or heart. As a rule, scleroderma is worse in blacks (especially black women) and in those who develop it after the age of forty-five.

Unfortunately, no cure exists for scleroderma, and treatment is largely directed at alleviating the symptoms. Raynaud's phenomenon is managed by the commonsense recommendation to wear proper gloves at all times when outdoors in cold weather and by the prescription of such blood vessel-dilating agents as prazosin, nifedipine, and topical nitroglycerine. Dryness and irritation of the skin must also be prevented by the regular use of strong emollients (such as **Lac-Hydrin** lotion) massaged in at least twice daily and by the use of mild detergents and cleansers (such as **Oil of Olay Sensitive Skin Bar**). Regular exercise is also encouraged to help maintain skin pliability. In severe cases the use of strong systemic agents such as penicillamine and colchicine are tried in an effort to soften the skin and decrease its thickness. Additional information may be obtained by contacting the United Scleroderma Foundation, 21 Brennan Street, Suite 21, P.O. Box 350, Washingtonville, California 95077.

Dermatomyositis

As indicated by its name, the skin and skeletal muscles are the primary sites of immunologic assault in dermatomyositis. In *polymyositis*, a closely related disorder, only the muscles are involved. Both conditions share the common feature of inflammatory immunologic damage to the muscles of the upper arms and upper legs. An underlying infectious viral process initiating the autoimmune reactions has been suggested as an underlying cause of at least some cases of these conditions.

In general, both dermatomyositis and polymyositis are more common in women than in men. The average age of onset for both is about fifty. In the beginning the symptoms tend to be subtle, and patients may note only some weakness in their upper arms and legs. With time, however, they experience increasing difficulty in rising from a chair or climbing stairs; eventually even such simple activities as combing their hair or raising their head from the pillow may prove too much for them. Those with dermatomyositis will additionally develop a peculiar lilac-colored discoloration on their eyelids and knuckles, known as the *heliotrope rash*.

The history and physical examination for dermatomyositis and polymyositis usually point to the diagnosis of these conditions. During the course of muscular inflammation, massive amounts of specific muscle tissue enzymes such as *creatine phosphokinase* (CPK) pour into the bloodstream, and this finding is very supportive evidence for the diagnosis. *Electromyography*, which are special tests in which small electrode needles are placed into the affected muscles to evaluate their function, can verify more subtle cases of muscle weakness and can also help select sites for muscle biopsies to confirm the diagnosis.

Oral corticosteroids are the mainstays of therapy. Moderate to high doses are usually given until muscle strength returns and muscle enzyme levels fall to normal, indicating suppression of inflammation. At times an additional potent agent, azathioprine (**Imuran**) may be needed. Happily, most patients make a full functional recovery, although many continue to have mild residual weakness of the shoulders and hips. In general, about 20 percent of patients require continued therapy five years after onset, but as many as 50 percent recover during that time. Unfortunately, relapses are possible.

Dermatomyositis and polymyositis have gotten a fair amount of media notoriety recently in regard to an alleged connection between these conditions and the use of the injectable filler substances **Zyderm** and **Zyplast** collagen, used for treating acne scars and wrinkles. Several individuals have claimed that the onset of their polymyositis was immunologically initiated by the collagen filler substance they received. Whatever the status of the litigation at this time, the medical evidence for these assertions seems wanting. To date no antibodies to native human collagen have been detected in individuals who have received **Zyderm** collagen, making the connection between the injected collagen and the dermatomyositis unlikely. And even when antibodies are detected, they are exclusively directed at the calf collagen-derived implant material. Discussing the safety issue, the American Rheumatologic Association said it has found that people treated with injectable collagen do not have a higher incidence of immunologically mediated disease. If anything, the incidence is less than expected. Moreover, a recent article on the subject in the respected *Journal of Dermatologic Surgery and Oncology* concludes: "There are no epidemiologic or scientific data to support the alleged link in the media and litigation between injectable bovine collagen material and dermatomyositis/polymyositis." To date over a million people have been treated with injectable collagen filler materials with relatively few problems, and the FDA continues to permit the marketing of these products for their approved uses.

AUTOIMMUNE THYROIDITIS

Autoimmune thyroiditis, also known as *Hashimoto's thyroiditis*, is a relatively common disorder caused by immune destruction of the thyroid gland, a small but vitally important gland that straddles the windpipe at the base of the front of the neck. The condition is most common in women and usually begins sometime between the ages of twenty and forty.

In the course of the disease Hashimoto's thyroiditis exhibits two main phases: a temporary phase of thyroid gland *over*activity and a permanent phase of *under*activity. The hyperthyroid phase is believed to be due to an excessive release of thyroid hormone (which is primarily responsible for regulating body metabolism) from the acutely immune-damaged gland. Persistent inflammation eventually results in the severely diminished thyroid output that marks the second phase of the disease.

Not surprisingly, the symptoms of autoimmune thyroiditis are essentially those of first acute *hyper*thyroidism (overactive metabolism) and later chronic *hypo*thyroidism (underactive metabolism). Individuals suffering with the problem typically develop a goiter (an enlarged, rubbery-feeling thyroid gland).

Endocrinologists (gland specialists) usually suspect the diagnosis of autoimmune thyroiditis from the history and physical examination. Two special autoantibody tests of the blood, the *antithyroglobulin antibody* and the *antimicrosomal antibody*, help to confirm the diagnosis. A biopsy of the thyroid gland may also be required.

Once the active inflammation has "burned out," thyroid hormone replacement therapy with medications such as **Synthroid** is the only treatment required. Periodic blood tests thereafter can assess drug dosage levels.

INSULIN-DEPENDENT (TYPE I) DIABETES MELLITUS

Insulin-dependent diabetes mellitus (IDDM) is a disease of reduced or completely absent insulin production caused by immune destruction of the insulin-secreting islet cells of the pancreas. Full progression usually occurs over a three-year period. Insulin is the hormone crucially involved in sugar regulation and usage in the body. Approximately ten thousand new cases of IDDM are reported each year. Until recently this condition was commonly called *juvenile-onset diabetes* because of the young ages at which it most often first appeared. Both genetic and environmental factors, particularly viral infections, have been implicated as possible contributing factors to the development of the disease. (IDDM must not be confused with the Type II variant, *adult-onset diabetes mellitus*, which results not from a lack of insulin but from an unexplained growing lack of tissue responsiveness with increasing age to the continued production of relatively normal amounts of insulin.)

The diagnosis of IDDM rests on the history and clinical examination and the finding of glucose intolerance, an inability to restore blood sugar levels to normal shortly after a high-sugar meal. A number of pancreatic islet cell autoantibodies, known collectively as *islet-cell surface autoantibodies*, have been identified in as many as 90 percent of patients, and these are used to help confirm the diagnosis in suspected individuals.

Treatment of IDDM consists largely of insulin replacement therapy to strictly control sugar metabolism. Recent evidence suggests that careful monitoring and strict control of blood glucose levels may actually reduce the risk of developing the many long-term complications of the disease such as heart disease, hypertension, blindness, nerve damage, and vascular insufficiency. Difficult cases often require the expertise of diabetologists, who are endocrinologists that specialize in diabetes care.

Two immune-suppressing agents, azathioprine (**Imuran**) and cyclosporine (**Sandimmune**), have been shown to induce remission in certain patients with IDDM, especially if administered within six weeks of initial diagnosis. Exactly how long such remissions will last needs further investigation, and it is believed that chronic therapy will usually be required. But whatever the long-term benefits of current medications, hope exists that newer immune-regulating agents and therapies will be even more effective in bringing about and maintaining long-term remissions.

ALOPECIA AREATA

Alopecia areata is a hair-loss condition in which oval or round bald spots appear. The characteristic finding under the microscope of scores of attacking lymphocytes surrounding the roots of the hair follicles in affected areas has suggested an autoimmune basis for this common condition. With as many as 20 percent of cases having a family history of the disorder, genetics is generally believed to play at least some role. Although hair loss per se is not a medically harmful condition, the emotional toll of alopecia areata cannot be underestimated.

While the scalp is most often affected, any hair-bearing site may be involved, including the beard, armpits, and genital area. Hair loss may occur gradually over one to three weeks or literally overnight. One or more completely hairless, smooth, and ivory patches may develop, ranging from one inch to five or more inches in diameter. Tapering hairs resembling exclamation marks may be seen at the edge of these patches. These "exclamation point" hairs are highly characteristic of alopecia areata and are extremely helpful to dermatologists for clinically diagnosing the condition. New bald patches may appear for several months. *Ophiasis* is the special name given to alopecia areata when it occasionally develops as a broad bald patch over an ear.

In about 5 percent of cases, alopecia areata progresses slowly to *alopecia totalis*, the complete loss of scalp hair. A much smaller percentage goes on to lose all body hair, including the eyebrows and eyelashes, a condition known as *alopecia universalis*. For some reason, as many as one out of every five sufferers also develops fingernail pitting.

In the vast majority of victims with limited involvement, the outlook for complete recovery is excellent. Future episodes are common, however, and occur in as many as one-third of the cases. In general, the earlier the onset of the condition and the more severe or extensive the episode, the worse the prognosis for complete regrowth.

Diagnosing alopecia areata seldom presents a problem. When your doctor has some question, however, a biopsy (a small removal of scalp tissue under local anesthesia) may be recommended. Monthly injections of antiinflammatory corticosteroids (for example, **Kenalog** suspension) directly into the affected areas are the mainstay of therapy in adults. High-potency topical steroid creams or ointments (**Ultravate**, **Temovate**, or **Diprolene**) applied twice daily are also often prescribed and are usually the treatment of choice in children with the condition. The absorption of topicals may be enhanced by placing them under occlusion, that is, by covering with a shower cap, **Saran Wrap**, or **Actiderm** dressing. Rarely prescribed because of their potential for side effects when used for long periods, oral corticosteroids are reserved for the most severe or resistant cases.

Various other topical irritants and allergens, including poison ivy resin, anthralin, dinitrochlorobenzene (DNCB), and aquaric acid dibutyl ester, have been used through the years to stimulate hair regrowth, with variable success. No one knows for sure how they work. Topical minoxidil lotion (**Rogaine**), currently used for treating certain forms of male and female pattern baldness, has also demonstrated some success in this condition. For more information you can contact the National Alopecia Areata Foundation, 714 C Street, Suite 216, San Rafael, California 94901.

VITILIGO

Vitiligo is another presumed autoimmune condition. In this disease the targets of attack are the skin's *melanocytes*, the pigment-producing skin cells. As in the case of alopecia areata, the psychological and social consequences of this disorder, especially in blacks exhibiting widespread involvement, cannot be minimized.

Affecting 1 percent of the American population, vitiligo is not rare. The disorder appears to run in some families, and many cases begin in childhood. Not long ago, vitiligo received quite a bit of media attention when black rock singer Michael Jackson announced that he was suffering with the condition.

Vitiligo may affect any area of the skin. The face, neck, nostrils, nipples, genitals, and other body-fold regions are favored locations. As a rule, pigment loss tends to be symmetrical: If the right side of the mouth loses color, the left usually does, too. In extensive cases, sufferers can be left with disfiguring zebra stripe-like patterns. Naturally, the darker the sufferer's normal skin tone, the more obvious the contrast between the affected and nonaffected areas.

The course of vitiligo is variable. Typically, periods of marked disease progression alternate with intervals of quiescence. Although repigmentation does occur occasionally on its own, complete spontaneous improvement is unfortunately rare.

For the experienced dermatologist, the diagnosis of vitiligo is obvious. In contrast to other depigmenting conditions, patches of vitiligo, when exposed to a Wood's ultraviolet light, demonstrate a stark white absence of all pigment. In uncertain cases a biopsy may be performed. The finding of a complete absence of melanocytes confirms the diagnosis.

Unfortunately, there is still no cure for vitiligo. Skin dyes (**Vitadye** and **Dyoderm**) and waterproof masking cosmetics (**Covermark** and **Dermablend**) can be satisfactory for hiding small areas of involvement. For selected cases of more extensive involvement, oral or topical use of *psoralens* combined with periodic exposure to ultraviolet A radiation, a process known as PUVA (*p*soralens plus UVA), may be helpful. In extreme cases the few remaining normal-pigmented islands of skin can be completely and permanently depigmented by the repeated application of monobenzyl ether of hydroquinone (**Benoquin**). For more information about vitiligo, you may contact the National Vitiligo Foundation, Inc., Texas American Bank Building, P.O. Box 6337, Tyler, Texas 75711.

CHAPTER THIRTEEN

WHEN FIRST AID REALLY COUNTS: ANAPHYLAXIS

Although you may find them uncomfortable or annoying, most allergy attacks do not require emergency first-aid measures or dramatic medical intervention. Simple itchy rashes in most instances are satisfactorily treated by the avoidance of the culprit allergen and the brief use of topical antiinflammatory creams and oral antihistamines. Respiratory allergies, such as those related to pollens and house dust, can also be managed most of the time by allergen avoidance (whenever possible) coupled with the use of oral antihistamines, decongestants, and inhalants. While these kinds of allergic reactions can be managed by relatively simple measures, a specific type of allergic reaction known as anaphylaxis is, by contrast, a potentially lethal medical emergency that requires immediate first-aid measures and often hospitalization.

In Chapter 1 you learned that previously sensitized (that is, allergic) individuals possess an overabundance of IgE allergen-specific antibodies, the particular antibodies responsible for immediate hypersensitivity (rapid-onset allergy) reactions. You may also recall that these antibodies typically attach themselves to the surfaces of both the basophils and the mast cells (the special cells that store many of the chemical substances responsible for allergic symptoms), which are found in most tissues of the body as well as in the bloodstream. During a typical allergy attack, allergens bind to the cell-surface-bound IgE molecules, causing them to release the potent chemical mediators responsible for producing allergy symptoms.

Anaphylaxis is the term used to describe the acute and dramatic signs and symptoms that can be triggered by some IgE-allergen interactions. When an IgE-mediated reaction is confined to a relatively small area, such as the mucous membranes of the nose and throat in the case of seasonal or perennial rhinitis, we call the reaction *local anaphylaxis*. On the other hand, when an allergen is absorbed, ingested, or injected into the body, severe and often life-threatening *systemic* (body-wide) symptoms may follow within seconds to minutes. For some people the rapidly ensuing symptoms may include a profound drop in blood pressure as well as heart and lung failure. When this type of response occurs, the reaction is known as *generalized anaphylaxis*.

As a rule the specific signs and symptoms of anaphylaxis are very much the same from one episode to another in the same individual. However, the particular manifestations may differ sharply from one person to the next. In other words, one person's anaphylactic symptoms are not necessarily identical to those of another. Most of the clinical manifestations are believed to be due to a widespread massive release of histamine as well as other chemicals that promote leaky blood vessels throughout the body and a narrowing of the airways.

The classic symptoms of anaphylaxis include any combination of the following: itching, flushing, small and giant hives, and a precipitous drop in blood pressure accompanied in some cases by a markedly increased heart rate or, less often, a severe slowing of the heart. Other well-known manifestations include shortness of breath, wheezing (difficulty exhaling), stridor (difficulty inhaling due to swollen vocal cords), intestinal and uterine cramping, vomiting, and diarrhea (sometimes bloody). Before going into shock, many victims commonly describe a feeling of impending doom.

Anaphylaxis may be triggered by an ever-growing list of frequently encountered chemical agents and substances. Foods, particularly shellfish and peanuts, are well-known causes. Other kinds of nuts and seeds have likewise been responsible for a number of fatalities, especially when susceptible individuals have consumed items that contain hidden ground nuts, such as cookies, candies, and pastries. Additionally, a wide variety of other foods and food additives, including legumes, celery, fish, eggs, grains, milk, aspartame (**NutraSweet**), sulfites (common food and beverage preservatives), and monosodium glutamate (a flavor enhancer), have also been found to trigger anaphylaxis in susceptible individuals.

Drugs and biological substances, like insulin, which the body makes, but which doctors may administer from outside sources, are also common triggering factors. Of these, the most common cause of anaphylactic shock is injected penicillin. Others include aspirin; insulin, either animal-derived or even the newer genetically engineered "human" insulin; antibiotics; local and general anesthetics; chemotherapeutic agents, such as those used in cancer treatment; enzymatic agents, such as those in papain (found in meat tenderizers and also used to treat certain gastrointestinal disorders); chymotrypsin (which is used for dissolving herniated spinal cord disks); blood products for transfusion; gamma-globulin; allergy extracts used for desensitization shots (allergy shots); and latex proteins in examining gloves and condoms. Snorting cocaine has also been associated with it. And last but far from least, insect stings are perhaps the most dramatic and well-known cause of anaphylaxis. Occurring in somewhere between 0.5 percent and 5 percent of the general population, sting-related anaphylaxis has been the most extensively studied of all varieties.

Exercise-induced anaphylaxis is a special, relatively uncommon form of the problem in which episodes are precipitated by vigorous exercise, especially in those with a history of asthma, hay fever, or eczema. Sometimes these attacks follow the eating of certain foods, such as celery or shellfish, which suggests but does not prove that there is an association between the consumption of these dietary items and vigorous exercise in the causation of the condition. Finally, there is a small group of sufferers in whom an exhaustive search for a triggering culprit of any kind, immunologic or otherwise, comes up empty. Doctors refer to this special category as *idiopathic anaphylaxis* or anaphylaxis of unknown cause. Regardless of the lack of clear-cut triggering factors, the signs and symptoms of idiopathic anaphylaxis do not differ from those of ordinary anaphylaxis.

Anaphylactoid (literally, anaphylaxislike) reactions are a related category of adverse reactions. While the clinical picture of anaphylactoid reactions is indistinguishable from the anaphylactic reactions just described, no IgE antibodies are found. For that reason a purely allergic basis for this problem is believed unlikely. Moreover, unlike true allergies, anaphylactoid reactions may occur on first exposure to a substance, whereas allergy attacks require prior exposure and a period of sensitization (a kind of "incubation" period) to the triggering allergenic agent. As of now, anaphylactoid reactions have been linked most commonly to the administration of iodine-containing X-ray contrast material and to the ingestion of certain nonsteroidal antiinflammatory drugs.

Diagnosing anaphylactic reactions is usually not difficult. The manifestations generally appear rapidly, within seconds to minutes after exposure to the provoking agent, and they typically progress with frightening rapidity. Following treatment, doctors may confirm their suspicions about the possible allergic cause(s) in a patient by the use of intradermal skin testing to suspected culprits or by the RAST, looking for abnormally elevated levels of IgE antibodies in the blood. They may also elect to perform a *basophil histamine release test*, another blood test, which examines allergen-triggered, IgE-mediated release of histamine from the basophils. When these tests indicate an allergic basis for the reaction, doctors say the tests are positive. Unfortunately, not all suspected allergens are available for testing at this time, limiting the usefulness of these examinations.

The importance of consultation with an allergist or immunologist following an episode of anaphylaxis cannot be overemphasized. Clearly, discovering what to avoid whenever possible is in itself a life-saving measure of the utmost importance, and once this has been determined, wearing a **Medic Alert** necklace or bracelet listing the substance(s) to which you are allergic is another critical step. For more information you may contact Medic Alert Foundation, P.O. Box 1009, Turlock, California 95380. At the very least a medical emergency card stating the history of anaphylaxis and its presumed causes should be carried in your wallet or purse at all times.

FIRST-AID AND EMERGENCY MEDICAL CARE

Avoidance of any known or potential triggering agent is of course the best of all possible ways to deal with anaphylaxis. Should an attack occur despite all preventive measures, however, it is critical to remember that *anaphylaxis is a medical emergency in which minutes count.* Once it starts, there is precious little time to lose! Emergency medical assistance must be started without delay, and emergency assistance must be summoned immediately since loss of consciousness can follow quickly without much warning.

For an attack in progress, epinephrine (**Adrenalin**) is the drug of choice and must be administered right away. It works by stopping the release of the chemicals responsible for the reaction. For this reason anaphylaxis-prone individuals should keep with them at all times an epinephrine emergency self-administration injectable kit (such as **EpiPen** and **Ana-Kit**). Naturally, they as well as their families should thoroughly familiarize themselves with the contents of these kits and their correct use beforehand. An anaphylactic attack is no time to begin learning what to do.

Ana-Kit (made by Hollister-Stier, Spokane, Washington) contains a syringe and needle preloaded with two doses of epinephrine. The device possesses a plunger lock rigged to prevent administering more than one doseful at a time. The kit also contains chewable antihistamine tablets (chlorpheniramine), alcohol swabs, and a tourniquet. For those unwilling or unable to self-administer the injections, **EpiPen** (manufactured by Center Laboratories, Port Washington, New York) is a good alternative. These kits contain a spring-loaded injector that automatically injects a preset dosage; the mechanism is tripped when the tip is pressed firmly against the user's skin. The company also makes **EpiPen Junior** for use in small children. As a rule epinephrine injections may be repeated every fifteen or twenty minutes until help arrives.

In the case of insect sting anaphylaxis, applying an ice pack or cold compress may retard the absorption of the venom and slow the progress of the reaction somewhat. The use of a tourniquet may also help do this and should be applied above the sting, in the direction in which blood returns to the heart. Remember to loosen the tourniquet for one minute every three minutes in order to prevent serious permanent tissue damage from prolonged, excessively diminished blood flow.

Once the individual is at the hospital, doctors may initiate other forms of therapy as needed. These may include the use of systemic antihistamines, such as diphenhydramine (**Benadryl** or **Atarax**) and corticosteroids such as prednisone or dexamethasone. Since the onset of action of corticosteroid agents generally takes several hours, these medications are of little use in the first-aid setting. Once they begin to work, however, they are especially important for controlling later stage symptoms. They are also useful as preventive therapy, especially in people who have experienced repeated episodes of idiopathic anaphylaxis. In cases of a severe blood pressure drop or respiratory problems, doctors may also need to institute intravenous fluid replacement, blood pressure-elevating drugs and oxygen therapy. Intubation (placing a tube through the mouth into the trachea) and other respiratory support measures may also be required. Fortunately, when first-aid measures are instituted early, the prognosis for complete, uncomplicated recovery is excellent.

CHAPTER FOURTEEN

HOCUS-POCUS AND SNAKE OILS: WATCH OUT FOR ALLERGY QUACKERY

So many different conditions and diseases of one kind or another have been ascribed by the lay public to allergies these days that the diagnosis and treatment of allergic disorders have made particularly fertile ground for the growth of medical quackery. Since a great deal of heated controversy generally surrounds the value and even the medical legitimacy of alternative or unconventional treatments in managing allergic conditions, it is important to examine some of these issues. Misinformation and misguided treatments can be not only costly but cause the loss of your life.

The word quack is derived from the term "quacksalver," which literally means to "quack like a duck about one's own salves and remedies." A congressional committee that recently looked into quackery defined it as "the practices and pretensions of a quack," and a quack was defined as "anyone who promotes medical schemes or remedies known to be false, or which are unproven, for a profit."

Not surprisingly, promotionalism—that is, advertising and publicity for the sake of making money—is at the heart of most allergy-related quackery. In some instances the information contained in advertisements or "infomercials" is merely intentionally misleading, but at other times it may be downright false. Admittedly more difficult to recognize yet sometimes no less misleading information comes from poorly researched articles found in widely read newspapers or trendy magazines. And perhaps the most difficult to recognize variety comes in the form of radio and TV talk show appearances by self-proclaimed experts and other health gurus with undisclosed financial interests in the therapies or treatments they are hawking. This form of "hidden advertising" is potentially the most dangerous, and we must all be on our guard against it.

WHAT MAKES ALLERGY QUACKERY THRIVE?

If promotion for profit is the seed of allergy quackery, confusion is the medium in which it grows and thrives. For one thing, the general public believes that allergies of all kinds are much more widespread problems than scientific evidence so far has shown. In a random sampling of some thirty-three hundred Americans, more than 40 percent believed that they possessed a true allergy to certain foods. Experts maintain, however, that the incidence of true immune-mediated allergies in the population at large does not exceed 2 percent of the population. It has been suggested that intense media attention to such issues as toxic dump sites, PCB (polychlorinated biphenyls) contamination, and Agent Orange-related conditions in Vietnam veterans (among other environmental concerns) have contributed to heightened public fears about allergies as well. For the average citizen, allergies, like these other conditions, seem to be shrouded in a certain mystery.

Because they are sometimes hard to pin down or are the result of a variety of complex factors, certain kinds of symptoms lend themselves to exploitation by allergy quacks. Without question there are many truly allergy-related conditions, as this book is ample evidence, but at the same time a substantial number of supposed "allergy" symptoms and disorders actually result from nonimmunologic mechanisms or even psychological causes. For example, as already discussed, some so-called food allergies do not involve the immune system at all and are in fact intolerances rather than allergies. For example, an intolerance to milk or milk products (lactose intolerance) is not an allergy to these products, as many people believe; instead it is an inherited enzyme deficiency that affects as many as 10 percent of adults.

In a similar vein, when asked whether they are allergic to antibiotics or aspirin, many people who have experienced headaches, upset stomachs, or yeast vaginitis when taking these medications will erroneously respond, for want of proper information, that they are "allergic" to the drugs when in fact their reactions are some of the common, nonallergic side effects of these agents. Such a climate of misinformation and lack of information is the perfect setting for quack doctors and quack remedies to flourish.

PHONY DIAGNOSTIC TESTING

If misinformation makes people more vulnerable to quacks and quackery, a variety of phony diagnostic tests puts them completely at the mercy of their exploiters. Through the years nonconventional practitioners have joined forces with some office laboratory suppliers to market a number of bogus allergy tests and testing procedures. In the area of tests, the American Academy of Allergy and Immunology has focused on five controversial ones that are not only of dubious scientific or medical value but in certain cases have proven themselves harmful or even fatal:

1. *Cytotoxic testing* or *Bryan's Test* heads the list. Performed in one of two ways, cytotoxic testing is a supposed method for detecting food allergies in particular. Less commonly, the test is performed *in vivo*—that is, using the patient as the testing ground. First the patient consumes a sample of the suspected food culprit, and then a blood sample is taken to look for either physical changes in the white blood cells or a fall in their absolute number. More commonly the test is performed *in vitro*—in a test tube. Using a special test kit designed specifically for a physician's

office, a small amount of the suspected food allergen is added to a sample of the patient's blood, once again looking for changes in the quality or quantity of the white cells.

Although admittedly the logic of these tests is appealing, the results of both kinds of cytotoxic testing proved so inaccurate in either confirming or excluding allergies that in the 1980s insurance carriers stopped reimbursing altogether for their use. In addition, not long afterward, the FDA banned the sale of the test kits entirely.

2. *The Rinkel method* is another dubious approach to evaluation and treatment of allergies. Otherwise known as the *skin titration* or *the intradermal titration approach,* this technique was used by some allergists for diagnosing suspected inhalant allergies (hay fever, dust, and dander problems) and for determining the lowest possible dosages to be used for allergy (desensitization) shots to subsequently treat them. The examination, which consists of skin testing with small, varying quantities of allergens, often arrives at treatment dosages that are actually much too low to be of any value in desensitizing against the allergens. The reverse is in fact true: Progressively increasing doses of allergens are generally needed to evoke the immune responses necessary to blunt IgE allergy attacks. Even in the case of maintenance shots, it has been found that the higher the dose, the greater the relief.

3. *Subcutaneous provocative and neutralization testing* has likewise fallen into disrepute in recent years. Similar to the Rinkel method, subcutaneous provocative testing consists of injecting suspected food allergens into the skin in varying quantities in an attempt to find the lowest dose of allergen needed to suppress or "neutralize" the patient's symptoms. Once the "appropriate" dose is determined in this fashion, weekly or twice weekly injections are maintained thereafter with the stated expectation of continuing to "neutralize" the patient's allergy symptoms.

4. *Sublingual provocative and neutralization tests* differ from the subcutaneous variety only in that the food allergens used in the former (administered in the form of liquid extracts) are in this case

placed under the tongue rather than injected into the skin. Nevertheless, like the former, this test, too, has proven of no value. At the same time, both tests pose a considerable risk to the patient, having at times been found to precipitate life-threatening anaphylaxis in individuals possessing true food allergies.

5. *Autogenous urine immunization*, also known as *urine autoinjection*, is likewise frowned upon these days. In vogue several decades ago, this method for diagnosing and treating allergies consists of injecting the patient's own urine into his skin. The theory behind the technique is about as scientifically spurious as the method is unappealing to the psyche. Not surprisingly, the technique is also potentially dangerous since we know that laboratory rabbits injected experimentally with their own urine developed severe kidney disease.

You should be equally wary of three other diagnostic procedures that may still occasionally be recommended by some practitioners:

1. *Applied kinesiology* is a chiropractic method that tests muscular strength reactions to suspected allergens in a variety of unproven ways.
2. *Radionics* uses electronic devices to measure "energy."
3. *Medical dowsing* uses a pendulum or dowsing (literally, divining) rods for this purpose.

If you encounter any practitioner who suggests these tests or procedures to you, you would be well advised to seek treatment elsewhere.

CLINICAL ECOLOGY

Clinical ecology is a medically unrecognized subspecialty that was originated more than twenty years ago by Theron Randolph, a physician, and his wife. Adherents of this approach maintain that a host of common physical and emotional disorders are actually triggered in susceptible individuals by long-term, low-level exposures to certain foods or chemicals. These conditions have been variously and sometimes fancifully termed by clinical ecologists "environmental illness," "ingestion intolerance," "cerebral (brain) allergy," "food addiction," or the "total allergy syndrome." In effect, patients are told that they are allergic to the "twentieth century" or to "everything modern." Interestingly, in 1971, Theron diagnosed the condition in himself and his wife and won a suit against the United States Internal Revenue Service for reimbursement of money spent for "organically grown" foods to treat their condition.

Nevertheless, since that time validation of clinical ecology has not been forthcoming from other sources. Based on a lack of scientific and clinical data, in 1981 the California Medical Association (CMA) adopted the position that the field of clinical ecology did not constitute a valid medical discipline. In 1984 a CMA task force, commissioned in response to protests by clinical ecologists, concluded as follows:

(1) There is no convincing evidence that supports the hypotheses on which clinical ecology is based; (2) clinical ecologists have not identified specific, recognizable diseases caused by exposure to low environmental stressors; (3) methods to diagnose and treat such unidentified conditions have not been shown to be effective; (4) the practice of clinical ecology can be considered experimental only when its practitioners adhere to scientifically sound research protocols and inform their patients about the experimental nature of their practice.

More recently these sentiments were echoed by both the American Academy of Allergy and Immunology and the American College of Physicians.

Research findings suggest that many of the so-called cases of environmental or food-related illness have a large psychological component. In one study involving twenty-six individuals who had been diagnosed as having environmental illness, investigators found that nearly two-thirds met the objective diagnostic criteria for mood and anxiety disorders. Similarly, in another study of plastics industry workers, it was found that many of those who developed environmental illness scored higher on objective tests for the presence of psychological disease.

If the validity of clinical ecology is in doubt, does this necessarily mean that the whole notion of environmental illness should be discarded entirely? For the moment I believe the answer is no. But until more information is available, we must maintain a healthy skepticism about the subject.

CANDIDIASIS HYPERSENSITIVITY SYNDROME

For more than a decade some physicians, most notably William Crook and C. O. Truss who popularized the idea, have been blaming a multitude of symptoms ranging from headache, chronic fatigue, irritability, inability to concentrate, gastrointestinal upset, hyperactivity and emotional disorders on overexposure and underlying allergy to the common yeast organism *Candida albicans*. The notion of "yeast hypersensitivity" was intellectually attractive and, as so often happens in these cases, was quickly picked up and disseminated by the popular press. Hence was born the much-talked-about "yeast connection."

There is absolutely no question that *candida*, or monilia, as it is also sometimes called, can cause us medical problems. Normally colonizing the gastrointestinal tract, *candida* is generally kept from overgrowing and causing any problems by the presence of certain bacteria with which it maintains a delicate balance of coexistence. However, when this equilibrium is upset, as for example by the use of antibiotics, estrogen, or birth control pills, the result is often the itching, burning, and discharge associated with garden-variety yeast vaginitis, which in most cases is easily treated by withdrawing the predisposing medications and treating with topical and/or oral antiyeast medications, specifically nystatin, terbenafine, and ketoconazole (**Mycostain**, **Lamisil**, and **Nizoral**).

On the other hand, when it comes to the so-called yeast hypersensitivity syndrome, the matter is not so straightforward. For one thing, the symptoms ascribed to the syndrome are vague and may be caused by many other physical or psychological diseases. Therefore, definitively diagnosing the condition by history is difficult, to say the least. Secondly, no specific tests are currently available to specifically diagnose the syndrome. Even the yeast skin tests and stool culture examinations often recommended by proponents of the "yeast connection" are actually of little value, since more than 90 percent of the general population will have a positive test.

To date, the jury is not yet in on the actual merits of the "yeast connection" or whether it is even a real entity. What we can say is that at present the available medical evidence offers little support for it. In a recent study a group of women with symptoms that have been ascribed to yeast hypersensitivity were divided into two groups. One group received nystatin (the antiyeast drug most commonly prescribed for the condition) orally and the other group received a placebo. Investigators found no difference in the overall success rate of treatment, casting further doubt on the whole yeast-allergy hypothesis.

Fortunately, nystatin, yeast elimination diets, and the environmental modifications often recommended by clinical ecologists to treat the syndrome are not by themselves necessarily harmful. It is more likely that when hosts of unnecessary and expensive tests are ordered and unproven treatments are advised that real problems will arise. Most important, if there is a more critical underlying condition that is causing the symptoms, serious consequences may result from the delay in seeking proper treatment.

"HOPE IN A BOTTLE"

When it comes to developing skin allergies to something you apply to your skin , there is a good rule of thumb: The more ingredients the product contains, the greater the chance you have of developing an allergy to it. For this reason I have chosen to include a word of caution in this chapter on allergy quackery about purchasing certain kinds of cosmetics.

Many years ago Charles Revson, the founder of Revlon Cosmetics, commented that the cosmetics industry sells "hope in a bottle." And probably nowhere in the cosmetics world is that more evident than in the $2 billion moisturizer market. You have moisturizers and lubricants that claim to be "antiaging," "antiwrinkling," "deep energizing," "nourishing," "pore-shrinking," "cellular-activating," "cellular-repairing," "skin-firming," and "cellulite-removing," to name just a few of the more common Madison Avenue ploys to get you to buy what in most cases amounts to little more than a fancy cold cream. To this basic formulation some manufacturers add one or more ingredients that are supposedly responsible for their product's many miracles, including collagen, pro-collagen, elastin, amino acids, algae, vitamin E (tocopherol), vitamin A, hyaluronic acid, DNA, RNA, allantoin, placental extract, eggs, milk, honey, and royal bee jelly. The chicanery here is not in hawking phony diagnostic tests, suggesting illnesses, or offering bogus treatments but in promoting products with lots of unnecessary ingredients that really do little or nothing for you except expose you to an increased potential risk for developing skin allergies to the additives. Unfortunately, the problem of unnecessary ingredients is by no means limited to moisturizers and may be found in many other kinds of cosmetics. For this reason you would do well to keep in mind another good rule: *Caveat emptor* (let the buyer beware).

CONCLUSION

Perhaps a 1993 medical article on allergy quackery in a recent issue of *New York State Journal of Medicine* devoted exclusively to health fraud summarizes the issue best:

Allergy-related quackery is a serious problem with powerful psychological, social, and economic implications which favor its perpetuation. Health professionals, third-party payers, lawmakers, regulatory agencies, the courts, and consumer groups must come together on the common ground of endorsing only sound scientific health care to curtail abuses and help patients find effective care.

The best means of finding a competent physician is by asking your family practitioner, pediatrician, or internist for a referral. If you do not have a primary doctor, you may contact your local or county medical society for a list of recommendations. As in choosing any physician, you would do well to consult a board-certified specialist, preferably one who holds a professorial teaching position at the largest local medical center in your area. Because of their active involvement in teaching and research, such physicians usually practice the most up-to-date medicine. For the diagnosis and treatment of inhalant allergies and asthma, you may also contact the American Academy of Allergy and Immunology, 611 East Wells Street, Milwaukee, Wisconsin 53202. For skin allergies, you might want to get in touch with the American Academy of Dermatology, P.O. Box 4014, Schaumburg, Illinois 60168.

COMMON ALLERGY TESTS

E ven in our high-tech world, there are still no adequate substitutes for the physician's complete medical history and thorough physical examination when dealing with any health problem. However, many times doctors must resort to a variety of testing procedures to diagnose or confirm allergic problems. The following is a summary of the more common tests used by doctors for diagnosing and evaluating allergy sufferers.

This is only an overview, of course, and is by no means a complete listing of all diagnostic examinations. It is intended only to supplement your physician's explanations, and your doctor may order additional tests as needed according to your particular problems. I have included only those tests that relate specifically to allergy and have excluded those routine tests, such as blood counts, liver and kidney function screens, and urine examinations, that are frequently done to be sure there are no underlying disorders responsible for your symptoms.

You should consult with your doctor concerning any questions you may have about any test. A description of the signs and symptoms and other details relating to the diagnosis of any of the conditions for which the following tests may be ordered can be found in the individual chapters devoted to them.

TESTS FOR IGE

IgE testing is used primarily for evaluating persons having nasal or chest symptoms suggestive of seasonal and perennial rhinitis and asthma. For that reason they are more strictly considered *confirmatory* tests rather than diagnostic tests. Two types of IgE tests are routinely performed: allergy skin tests and RAST.

Skin Tests

Skin testing is particularly useful for confirming dander, dust, mold, and pollen allergies. They are also useful for confirming penicillin allergy in persons who are unsure of whether they are indeed allergic to penicillin and for whom penicillin (or its derivatives) would be the best form of treatment for their condition.

Skin testing can be accomplished in two ways. One method, *scratch tests*, consists of placing the test material over a small scratch or puncture in the skin. Alternatively, with *intradermal tests*, the allergens are injected directly into the superficial skin. Depending on the number of allergens tested, twenty or more scratches or sticks are ordinarily required. Because they are performed on the living body, both types of skin tests are categorized by doctors as *in vivo* testing.

A positive test—that is, a reaction that confirms the presence of IgE antibodies—consists of the appearance of an itchy, raised, reddish hive appearing at the test site within minutes of exposure to the allergen. In general the hive that forms resembles the kind seen as the result of an ordinary mosquito bite. When no reaction occurs, doctors say the test is negative—that is, you do not appear to be allergic to the test substance.

Intradermal tests are generally more sensitive than scratch tests. However, they also tend to yield a greater number of false positives. This means that for some people the tests sometimes have a positive reaction at the test site even though they do not develop allergy symptoms to the substance tested when exposed to it in their everyday world. For this reason doctors rely on their experience and exercise a great deal of judgment when interpreting these tests and determining the applicability of the findings to a particular patient.

One obvious drawback to either type of skin testing is the necessity for multiple skin pricks. Another is that certain medications, such as antihistamines, can interfere with the tests, and therefore you must inform your doctor if you have been taking any of these agents. A third and far more critical concern is the remote possibility of inducing a serious, life-threatening (anaphylactic) reaction to one of the injected allergens. This is the reason that these tests are generally performed in settings equipped for emergencies and that most physicians insist that you remain under observation for about half an hour after testing.

RAST

Another common test for IgE antibodies is known as the RAST, which stands for radio allergo sorbent test. In this method a serum sample (the fluid that remains when all the red and white blood corpuscles have been separated out) is used to detect levels of IgE antibodies to specific allergens by means of a highly sensitive technique called a radioimmunoassay. The radioactive markers from which the test draws its name make the antibody easy to measure. Performed outside the body, doctors refer to the RAST as in vitro testing (tests done in a test tube).

The main advantage of the RAST method is that it requires only one stick to draw the blood sample, an obvious plus when dealing with children, excessively apprehensive adults, or patients with widespread skin rashes that might interfere with the doctor's ability to read the test results accurately. In addition, because it is not performed in the skin, RAST poses absolutely no risk to the patient. It is also useful for monitoring changes in IgE antibody levels once appropriate treatment has begun. On the downside, it is generally not as sensitive as skin testing for confirming the presence of allergies. That means it may miss picking up some instances of true IgE allergies. It is also some-what more costly to perform than routine skin testing.

"Use" Tests

When it comes to skin allergies, particularly those to cosmetics, your doctor may not have to resort to fancy testing to determine the specific cause(s). Instead you may be instructed to carry out a "use" test, which is essentially a set of trial-and-error tests that you perform yourself at home.

For the sake of illustration, let's say that you have developed an allergy to a particular brand of beige foundation. The first thing you would do (after the allergy has completely cleared or has been treated) is to switch to another brand of beige foundation. If after three straight days of use you don't develop allergic symptoms to the new product, it is unlikely that you are allergic to the beige pigment, but you may be allergic to some other ingredients in the original cosmetic such as the fragrance(s) or the preservative(s) in it.

Now suppose you do develop the same allergy with the new beige foundation. This suggests that you are allergic to the beige color itself. Again, once the allergic reaction has completely cleared, you might switch to a different color of foundation and try it for three days. If no problems develop, you may continue to use that product thereafter. However, if the different color of foundation produces an allergic reaction, it suggests that you are allergic to one of the many ingredients that comprise the base (that is, the vehicle) of most brands of foundations (regardless of manufacturer).

Use tests have the advantages of being painless, convenient, and easy to perform, especially when only one or two product types, such as blushers or foundations, are the suspected culprits. On the other hand, when you have to experiment with a number of different types of products, use tests can become quite time-consuming and sometimes expensive. When this is the case, your dermatologist may recommend patch tests to determine the cause(s).

Patch Tests

When no specific product or ingredient appears to be the cause of your allergy, patch tests are often recommended. They may also be ordered to confirm suspected cases of allergic contact dermatitis in order to distinguish the problem from nonallergic causes of skin rash.

For patch test purposes, allergens are typically grouped together in a variety of ways. Each grouping is referred to as a "battery" or "test series." Depending on the individual circumstances, several different patch test series may be performed. For example, when contact allergy is suspected but no specific allergen has been pinpointed as the possible culprit, your doctor may patch-test you to the contents of what dermatologists call a "standard" or "screening" tray, which consists of a battery of the twenty allergens most frequently associated with contact allergy as determined by the North American Contact Dermatitis Group. Although this list is periodically reevaluated and substitutions and addenda made whenever necessary, you should be aware that no screening series can possibly cover all the many allergens found in our ever-changing cosmetics, industrial products, and so forth.

Should your doctor suspect that the cause of your dermatitis is one or more of the topical medications you have been using or your exposure to certain types of clothing or fabrics, she may elect to patch-test you to "specific" batteries of allergens rather than to the screening materials. For example, you may be tested for the chemicals contained in the "rubber and metal" or "therapeutic" series. Although there is some overlap between the contents of the standard tray and the specific trays, the use of the latter generally permits a more precise identification of the culprits involved.

In general, patch tests are fairly simple to perform. The materials to be tested are usually dissolved in a petroleum jelly base and then applied to a patch, a small piece of absorbent material. Patches are then fixed to the skin by a strip of nonallergic tape. In a variation of this method, the test materials are individually placed in a series of tiny circular aluminum wells (known as Finn chambers) and then taped to the test sites. The large area of the upper back is the most frequent site for testing. Occasionally the inside skin on the upper arms is used, especially if there is a rash on the back or when only a few allergens are being tested.

In general, patches are left in place for forty-eight hours. They are then removed and the skin sites directly underneath examined for any responses. In search of possible delayed reactions, the test sites are often reexamined twenty-four hours and then seventy-two hours later as well. A positive test result (meaning that the skin has reacted) is usually graded on a scale of 1 to 4, with the latter representing a severe reaction in response to the test substance. Common test reactions, mimicking the patient's allergic skin problem, include itching, redness, swelling, pimple formation, and blistering.

Patch testing is certainly a more scientific method than trial and error for determining the underlying culprit(s) in a case of presumed allergic contact dermatitis. Nevertheless, these tests are somewhat artificial in that they do not necessarily reproduce the many real-life factors such as sweating and skin maceration or the effect of repeated applications of a substance. In addition, testing on the thick skin of the back is not always an effective means of reproducing allergies to items such as eye cosmetics that are intended for use on the very thin skin of the lids.

Although minute concentrations of test substances are used in patch testing, there is a small risk when performing these tests of sensitizing the skin (that is, causing an allergy to develop) to one or more of the test materials. Despite these limitations, properly interpreted patch tests remain the best form of "proof" available for establishing the diagnosis of allergic contact dermatitis to a particular agent. For that reason they have become medicolegally important in many instances of occupationally associated skin allergy.

It is important to note that a positive reaction does not always indicate that the allergen used in the test is the cause of the current problem of contact dermatitis. It does suggest, though, that the individual somewhere in the course of his or her life developed a sensitivity to that ingredient. With this in mind the dermatologist must work closely with the allergy sufferer to determine the relevance of any patch test finding to the present problem.

Once patch testing has implicated a specific allergen, your doctor may be able to recommend suitable products that do not contain that allergen, as well as methods of avoiding future exposure. You may also be given the various synonymous chemical, cosmetic, and pharmaceutical names under which the culprit allergen masquerades on product labels. Just as important, you will be given the names of any of its chemical relatives that are also likely to provoke allergy symptoms.

When a specific product or only a small number of differing products are suspected of provoking the allergy, your doctor may opt to patch-test you directly to those items. To do this, a small amount of the test cosmetic—or, in the case of clothing, a moistened piece of the item's fabric—is patch tested in the usual fashion and then evaluated for allergic reactions at intervals of forty-eight, seventy-two, and ninety-six hours. Certain eye cosmetics and other products containing volatile ingredients that tend to evaporate quickly on skin contact are allowed to thoroughly dry before being taped to prevent a nonallergic irritation that could confuse the test.

When a particular product has been found to be the cause of the skin allergy, common sense would dictate that merely avoiding that product from then on would end the problem. Unfortunately, this is not always the case since many products, even those by competing manufacturers, share many of the same ingredients. For this reason your doctor may elect to contact the manufacturer to explain your problem and to request that samples of the individual ingredients be sent to him or her for use in patch testing. In this way, once you have determined the specific ingredients that trigger your symptoms, you can avoid future exposure by simply checking product ingredient labels before purchase. Cosmetic manufacturers that label their products "hypoallergenic" are generally more likely to be helpful in this regard and to comply with your doctor's request for assistance.

Photopatch Tests

A variation of the patch tests just described, known as photopatch tests, can be very useful for diagnosing instances of suspected photoallergic contact dermatitis, a condition in which exposure to light, usually ultraviolet light, interacts with the contact allergen to provoke skin allergy.

In photopatch testing the patch test materials are applied in duplicate, usually to the lower back or occasionally to the undersurface of the forearms, and taped in place with opaque paper. After twenty-four hours one side is uncovered, exposed to a light source for thirty minutes, and then recovered. Both sides are then examined twenty-four hours later.

If there is no reaction at either site, the test is considered negative altogether. If both sides show a reaction, the skin allergy is most likely to be an ordinary contact dermatitis (that is, one that does not need light to provoke it). Photoallergy is confirmed when the side that received the light irradiation demonstrates itching, swelling, redness, hives, or blistering while the other side does not. As in ordinary patch testing, the severity of the reactions are graded on a scale of 1 to 4, with 4 representing the most severe response.

COMMON ALLERGY MEDICATIONS AND TREATMENTS

Without question there is no better way to "treat" any disorder than preventing its occurrence in the first place. And perhaps to no class of conditions does this rule apply more than to allergic disorders where the trigger is some potentially avoidable troublemaker such as animal dander or poison ivy. Nevertheless, there are times when avoidance is impossible, and your doctor must prescribe a variety of therapies to deal with your troublesome allergy symptoms. The following is a description of some of the more commonly employed therapeutic modalities currently available. For specific management of particular conditions, you should consult the appropriate sections of the book. Your physician should of course be your ultimate resource for the details about all forms of treatment.

SODIUM CROMOLYN

Since prevention is my favorite therapy, I have chosen to begin with sodium cromolyn, a medication that can be helpful for preventing or minimizing the symptoms of certain forms of allergic reactions. Although the precise mechanism of its actions is still unknown, cromolyn basically works by blocking the release of histamine, one of the major mediators of allergic symptoms, as well as other allergy provokers, from mast cells and basophils (the storehouses of these substances). Apart from its effects on mediators, cromolyn may also have a slight direct antiinflammatory action.

What is important to note is that cromolyn is not effective once an allergy attack has already begun. For best results it should therefore be initiated a few weeks before the allergy season has gotten underway. It must also be used between four and six times a day every day in order to be effective. If the allergy problem is an ongoing one, as in the case of perennial allergic rhinitis, you must anticipate waiting several weeks before realizing any possible benefits from the use of the drug. Unfortunately, not everyone responds to cromolyn, and there is currently no way to predict who will benefit. Nevertheless, since it has shown itself to be a relatively safe medication (even for use during pregnancy), it is worth a try in many cases of nasal allergies and asthma. For use in eye allergies, cromolyn is marketed as **Opticrom**; for nasal allergies, **Nasalcrom**; and for asthma, **Intal**.

ANTIHISTAMINES

Antihistamines remain the workhorses of antiallergy therapy. Through the years they have proven their usefulness in managing all kinds of allergies: local, systemic, internal, and external (skin) allergies. Because they resemble histamine in their molecular shapes, antihistamines, as the name suggests, work by competing with histamine for binding at a number of different tissue sites, such as the capillaries, nerve cells, and muscle cells lining the breathing tubes.

To date there are seven major classes of antihistamines, each containing many different drugs. With such a wide selection of medications, if one does not work well or causes too many side effects, there are fortunately many others to turn to. The two best known examples of the class known as *ethanolamines* are diphenhydramine (**Benadryl** and **Benylin**) and clemastine (**Tavist**). Perhaps equally well known are the *alkylamines*, chlorpheniramine (**Chlor-Trimeton**) and brompheniramine (**Dimetane**). The *ethylenediamines* are best represented by tripelennamine (**Pyribenzamene**); the *piprazines* by hydroxyzine (**Atarax**); and the *piperadines* by cyproheptadine (**Periactin**). The *phenothiazines*, known mostly for their value in psychiatric therapies, are best represented in allergy management by methdilazine (**Tacaryl**).

Sleepiness is the most annoying side effect of most antihistamines, although **Chlor-Trimeton, Tavist,** and **Tacaryl** are generally tolerated somewhat better than the others in this regard. Nevertheless, the brochures inserted in these products warn of general coordination impairment and against driving or operating dangerous machinery while taking them. It should thus go without saying that alertness will be even more impaired if antihistamines are combined with alcohol consumption or the use of tranquilizers. On the other hand, the sleep-inducing properties of these drugs are often used to advantage when they are taken before bedtime. (In fact, most commercial sleep aid medications contain diphenhydramine, the antihistamine contained in **Benadryl** and **Benylin**.)

Two other common antihistamine caveats deserve note. Persons with a history of glaucoma and those with histories of prostate enlargement or inflammation should take these drugs only after checking with their doctors since the obstructive symptoms of these conditions may be worsened by these agents.

To counteract the grogginess induced by antihistamines, manufacturers often combine them with decongestant ingredients (see below), which have an "upper" effect in addition to their decongestant properties. Well-known examples of such combination products include **Contac, Ornade,** and **Dristan** capsules. Sometimes antihistamines are combined with acetaminophen (as in **Tylenol Allergy Sinus Medication**) to reduce the headaches, aches, and pains that accompany allergy attacks. Most combination products are available without a doctor's prescription. While combination products are convenient to use and may provide relief for some sufferers, they may not be as effective for others because they do not allow dosage flexibility of the individual ingredients. In other words, with these medications you may get too little of one drug and too much of another for your needs. By contrast, if you take an antihistamine, a decongestant, and an analgesic (pain reliever) separately, you are able to adjust the dose and the dosage schedule of each to precisely what you need to suppress your specific symptoms.

Three products—terfenadine (**Seldane**), astemizole (**Hismanal**), and loratadine (**Claritin**)—that belong to the seventh category of antihistamines, the *nonsedating antihistamines,* deserve special mention. All three have been shown to be effective for controlling symptoms when taken as directed without inducing grogginess in the vast majority of instances. **Claritin** and **Hismanal** have the advantage of being taken only once a day, although the former generally begins to work in a matter of hours while the latter usually requires about two weeks to achieve optimal effects. **Seldane** must be taken twice daily but seems to begin working somewhat sooner. All three are relatively expensive compared to most antihistamines, and both **Seldane** and **Hismanal** *must not be taken along with the antibiotic erythromycin, or the antifungal agent ketoconazole* (**Nizoral**) *since potentially fatal heart rhythm abnormalities have resulted from these combinations.* To date, no such adverse interaction has been reported with the use of **Claritin.** Overall, the safety profile of these medications when taken as directed is quite satisfactory, making them excellent first choices of allergy therapy for active working people.

Although antihistamines of all classes are somewhat helpful once an allergy attack is underway, they are far more effective if taken before an attack has begun. Doing so allows sufficient time for the antihistamine to bind to its tissue receptors before histamine is released. This means that if you are allergic to dogs and you know that you will be exposed to one later in the day, take your antihistamine beforehand.

DECONGESTANTS

Decongestants are another class of popular drugs used to treat allergy symptoms. Working by constricting blood vessels, they are useful for shrinking swollen mucous membranes and slowing runny noses due to colds and allergies. Unlike cromolyn and many of the antihistamines, however, decongestants are quite effective in managing allergy attacks in progress.

Decongestants are sold as systemic and topical agents, in both drops and spray formulations. In general the topical preparations are more effective than their oral counterparts. Most are available over the counter (OTC), meaning that they may be purchased without a doctor's prescription. Popular oral decongestants include two kinds of pseudoephedrine tablets (**Sudafed** and **Afrin**). Topicals for the nose include phenylephrine (**Neosynephrine**) and oxymetazoline (**Afrin** and **Neosynephrine 12 Hour**) and for the eyes, tetrahydrozoline (**Visine** and **Murine Plus**).

Decongestants are not without their potential side effects and must be used with caution. Since these drugs are all stimulants, they can sharply raise the blood pressure, speed the heart rate, and provoke headaches and jitteriness. For this reason, if you suffer with high blood pressure, diabetes, heart rhythm abnormalities, or thyroid problems or if you take certain antidepressants, you would do well to check with your doctor before using any of these drugs, including the topical forms that can be absorbed to some extent into the bloodstream, particularly through the conjunctiva of the eyes or the nasal mucous membranes.

Special caution is advised when using decongestants topically. They should be used only for a short time—three to five days at the most—to control symptoms because continued use after that may result in *rebound* nasal congestion, a troublesome condition that doctors call *rhinitis medicamentosa*. In this condition a vicious cycle is established whereby the topical decongestant becomes needed to alleviate the symptoms its own overuse is responsible for causing. To avoid this unhappy consequence, you should use decongestants only as directed and only for the length of time specified in the product instructions or by your doctor.

CORTICOSTEROIDS

Corticosteroids are hormonelike antiinflammatory drugs used widely in many medical specialties for treating a broad spectrum of problems. For allergy treatment they have proven invaluable therapy and are available for topical use in spray, lotion, cream, and ointment formulations (as sprays and inhalants for use in the respiratory tract; as injectables for local therapy of small allergic skin rashes; and in intramuscular, intravenous, and oral forms for systemic therapy). Corticosteroids should not be confused with the sex steroids, the muscle-building hormones taken illicitly by some competitive athletes and some health enthusiasts; the two types of steroid are not related.

The relative potencies of topical corticosteroids have been put into seven main groupings, ranging from the superpotent (Group I) to the most mild (Group VII). In general, ointments (petroleum jelly-based products), because they are more occlusive, tend to be more potent than creams containing the same ingredients in equal concentrations. For example, **Maxiflor** 0.05% ointment is a group II preparation, whereas **Maxiflor** 0.05% cream is a group III (less potent) formulation.

Examples of superpotent topical steroids used to treat tough allergic skin disorders include **Ultravate, Temovate,** and **Diprolene.** Intermediate potency products include **Elocon, Westcort,** and **Locoid,** and mild preparations, **Aclovate** and **Hytone 2.5%.** This list is by no means complete, and your doctor may choose from a wide variety of other topical steroids depending on the nature of your problem, the location of the condition, and the anticipated duration of therapy. For example, milder corticosteroids are generally chosen for the genital area and face because the thin skin of these regions is more likely to experience an adverse reaction than, say, the thicker skin of the back.

Although they may look deceptively like simple body lotions, cold creams, or petroleum jelly products, topical corticosteroids should not be taken for granted and used as such. As a rule, the greater the potency of the topical steroid and the more applied, the greater the likelihood of side effects. Consequently, their use should be supervised by an experienced physician.

Some of the more common side effects resulting from long-term indiscriminate or unsupervised topical steroid use may include permanent thinning and "aging" of the skin; loss or patchy lightening of the normal skin color; the formation of networks of "broken blood" vessels (actually permanently dilated blood vessels) on the cheeks, nose, and elsewhere on the face, neck, and chest; easy bruisability; and stretch marks. Prolonged and widespread use, particularly of the potent and superpotent topical steroids, owing to their more significant absorption through the skin, may occasionally lead to suppression of native steroid production by the adrenal glands. Such suppression renders the individual temporarily less able to handle physical and emotional stress without the need for corticosteroid supplementation therapy during times of crisis. Fortunately, most of the adverse side effects of these drugs, including adrenal gland suppression, are reversible once the medication is stopped.

Topical steroids in spray mist form have proven particularly useful for treating nasal allergic symptoms. The most common preparations currently available are beclomethasone (**Beconase AQ** and **Vancenase AQ**), triamcinolone (**Nasacort**) and flunisolide (**Nasalide**). All are best started about two weeks before the allergy season is in full swing and must be continued throughout the season three to four times daily for optimal effect. **Nasacort** is used only once daily. These drugs are rarely responsible for headaches, nose bleeds, or erosion or ulceration of the nasal mucous membranes, and in general they produce remarkably few side effects.

Systemic corticosteroids (those administered orally or by intramuscular or intravenous routes) are usually categorized according to their duration of action. Those having maximum biologic activity for between eight and twelve hours, such as cortisone and hydrocortisone preparations, are known as short-acting steroids. Those having effects in the range of twelve to thirty-six hours, such as prednisone and methylprednisolone (**Medrol**) are designated intermediate-acting, and those retaining biological activity for between thirty-six and fifty-four hours, such as dexamethasone and betamethasone formulations (**Decadron** and **Celestone**, respectively), are classed as long-acting.

For short-term therapy, especially when administered in low doses, systemic corticosteroids cause remarkably few side effects. These may consist of headache, upset stomach, and some fluid retention. On the other hand, prolonged use of high doses of systemic steroids has been associated with a host of adverse effects including elevation of blood pressure, gastric ulcer formation, fluid accumulation, weight gain, electrolyte abnormalities, menstrual irregularities, growth impairment in children, and psychological disorders. Doctors attempt to avoid or minimize the risk of these problems by switching to alternate-day doses rather than daily dosing to allow the body to rebound to normal on the off days. Finally, since blood sugar levels are increased by steroids, diabetics must be monitored especially carefully. But despite these limitations, systemic corticosteroids continue to prove themselves invaluable drugs for the management of many acute and chronic allergic and autoimmune disorders when used under strict medical supervision.

IMMUNOTHERAPY

Immunotherapy, otherwise known as *desensitization* or *allergy shots*, can be an effective means of controlling a number of different kinds of allergies, particularly the seasonal and perennial varieties. They are often considered when drug therapy has not been sufficiently effective in providing symptomatic relief, when medication side effects have proven intolerable, when symptoms are so debilitating that they interfere seriously with a person's work, play, or sleep, and when an allergy is chronic (long-lasting).

Desensitization shots attempt to make the body's immune system more "tolerant" (less reactive) to the offending allergen(s). The method involves injecting, at first, minute quantities of the allergen and then gradually increasing the amounts over periods ranging from days to weeks or months until a dose of allergen is reached at which continued periodic injections throughout the year or booster shots will prevent the outbreak of symptoms whenever the allergen is encountered. Maximum benefit often requires two to three years to achieve. Occasionally, when more rapid protection must be attained, allergists sometimes accelerate the schedule by administering several increasing doses in a single day or, alternatively, giving daily injections for several days in succession. Whatever the schedule, a successful end result is an increase in the production of protective (IgG) blocking antibodies that compete with the troublesome (IgE) allergy-producing antibodies to prevent them from triggering the release of histamine.

Ironically, the main risk of allergy injections is themselves provoking allergy attacks or even potentially life-threatening anaphylaxis. For this reason doctors generally insist that patients remain in their offices for observation for at least half an hour after an injection. However, such reactions rarely occur when doses are properly adjusted and are administered in slowly increasing amounts. Overall, the main drawbacks of desensitization are the expense entailed and the inconvenience involved in frequent doctor visits.

Unfortunately, immunotherapy does not cure allergies, nor is it uniformly successful in treating all allergic conditions. And even when successful, it may not entirely suppress all allergy symptoms. In certain instances, however, such as in the treatment of ragweed pollen allergy (hay fever), if given enough time to work, desensitization has been shown to be highly effective in as many as 80 percent of patients. It is also highly effective in minimizing the risk of death from insect venom allergies in susceptible persons.

To be sure, the past quarter century has witnessed enormous gains in the fields of allergy prevention, diagnosis, and treatment. [While few would argue that our current methods are not the be-all and the end-all in the field], most would agree that we are now capable of doing much to alleviate allergy suffering simply and relatively inexpensively. Ongoing research in the fields of dermatology, allergy, and immunology promises to yield even better and more efficient ways to prevent and deal with allergic disorders in the not-too-distant future.

INDEX

antigens. *See* allergens
antihistamines, 6, 10, 36, 44, 58–60, 72,
  92, 93, 108, 109, 113, 130, 134–37,
  150, 151, 170–71, 185
  general description of, 192–94
  list of, 21–22
anti-itch preparations, 89, 93, 134
antimalaria drugs, 149, 154
antinuclear antibody test (ANA titer),
  154, 158
applied kinesiology, 176
Apresoline, 81
aquaric acid dibutyl ester, 164
arachnids, 29, 128, 136, 137
ARM, 22
arthritic diseases, 153–60
aspartame, 67–68, 168
Aspergillus, 27, 28
aspirin, 49, 55, 76, 81, 83, 86–87, 91,
  154, 168, 174
astemizole, 22, 77, 78, 194
asthma, 45–61
  air pollution and, 140
  allergic (extrinsic), 49
  food allergies and, 65, 69
  linseed and attacks of, 41
  nonallergic (intrinsic), 49–52
astringents, 95
Atarax, 171, 193
atopic dermatitis, 110–13
atopic individuals, 65, 129, 136–37
Atrovent inhaler, 58
autogenous urine immunization, 176
autoimmune disorders, 152–65
autoimmune thyroiditis, 161
avocados, 63
Ayr, 23
azathioprine, 149, 160, 162
Azmacort, 59
azo dyes, 55
Azulfidine, 83

B lymphocytes, 4
bacitracin, 66, 81, 109
Bactrim, 82, 88, 151
baldness, 163–64
balsam of Peru, 106, 108

bananas, 63
barbiturates, 83
barrier creams, 98–99, 101, 108, 109
basophil histamine release test, 169
basophils, 5, 7, 8, 166
bath oil, 118
beclomethasone, 197
Beclovent, 59
Beconase, 24, 197
bedbugs, 135–36
bedding, 29–30, 32, 35, 36, 42, 135, 137
bee stings, 73, 128–31
Benadryl, 21, 130, 150, 171, 192, 193
Benoquin, 165
Benylin, 92, 192, 193
benzalkonium chloride, 122
benzocaine, 89, 93
benzoic acid, 108, 116
benzoyl peroxide, 109
benzyl alcohol, 122
benzyl benzoate, 35
BHA, 68, 122
BHT, 68, 122
Biogel gloves, 105
bird breeder's lung, 145, 146
birth control pills, 151, 178
bisulfite, 68
black-and-blue nodules, 81
blood problems from drugs, 85
blood transfusions, anaphylaxis from, 168
Brethine, 57
Bricanyl, 57
2-bromo-2-nitropropane-1, 121
brompheniramine, 192
bronchial asthma. *See* asthma
bronchitis, chronic, 140
bronchodilators, 56, 57–58
bronchospasm, 47, 50, 83
Bronkodyl, 56
bronopol, 116
Bryan's test, 174–75
bubble bath products, 118
Butazolidin, 55, 81, 86
butylated hydroxyanisole (BHA), 68, 122
butylated hydroxytoluene (BHT), 68,
  122
butyric acid, 108

DEET, 132
dehumidifiers, 33
delayed reactions (Type IV reactions),
  6–9, 81
Dermablend, 165
Dermaffin, 99
Dermaprene, 105
Dermashield, 99
dermatitis
  allergic contact, 81, 89, 90, 100–13,
    120–25
  exfoliative, 82
  irritant contact, 94–99, 119–20
  photoallergic contact, 82, 107–8, 147,
    149–50
dermatomyositis, 159–60
desensitization shots. See allergy shots
dexamethasone, 171, 198
dextromethorphan, 92
diabetes mellitus, insulin-dependent
  (Type I), 161–63
diazolidinyl urea, 121–22
dibucaine, 89
dicloxacillin, 82, 87
Dilantin, 78, 81, 83–85
Dimetane, 192
dimethylglyoxime, 103
dinitrochlorobenzene (DNCB), 164
3-diol, 121
diphenhydramine, 21, 93, 130, 150, 171,
  192, 193
Diprolene, 102, 164, 196
discoid lupus erythematosis, 154
diuretics, 77, 78, 151
DNCB, 164
dog allergies, 37, 38–39, 40
Dowicil 200, 117
dowsing, medical, 176
Dristan, 193
drug challenges, 90–91
drug fever, 83
drug interactions, 78
druglike reactions to foods, 63
drug reactions
  allergic, 79–93
  nonallergic, 75–79
Duricef, 81, 83, 87

dust, 26–27, 49, 110, 184
  proofing the house against, 34–36
Dyoderm, 165
dyspnea, 48

ecology, clinical, 176–78
eczema
  atopic, 110–11
  as drug reaction, 82
  food allergies and, 65, 69
  "housewife's," 99
  photoallergic, 150, 151
EDTA, 122
EIA, 50–51
EIB, 50–51
Elastryn, 105
electromyography, 159
elimination diets, 70–71, 74, 112, 179
Elimite, 134
Elixophyllin, 56
Elocon, 102, 124, 196
environmental allergies, 139–51
environmental illness, 176–78
eosinophils, 5, 8, 90
ephedrine, 58
epinephrine, 56, 73, 92, 130, 170–71
EpiPen, 73, 131, 170
EpiPen Junior, 171
epoxy resins, 150
erythema multiforme, 82
erythema nodosum, 82
erythromycins, 60, 78, 84, 91
estrogen, 106, 178
ethanolamines, 192
ethylenediamines, 192–93
ethylenediaminetetraacetic acid, 122
Eurax, 134
eustachian tubes, congestion of, 14, 15
Euxyl K-400, 122
exercise-induced anaphylaxis, 168
exercise-induced bronchospasm, 50–51
exfoliative dermatitis, 82
eyelid sensitivity, 117, 118, 122, 188

false positive results, 69
farmer's lung, 145–46
FD&C Yellow No. 5, 55, 68, 86

Feldene, 151
Finn chambers, 187
fire ants, 128
fixed drug eruptions, 82
flaxseed, 40–41
fleas, 134–35, 136
flunisolide, 197
flu vaccine, 80
foam rubber, 32
food additives, 49, 54, 66–68, 168
food allergies, 28–29, 62–74, 174
    atopic dermatitis and, 110, 112
foods
    anaphylaxis triggered by, 167–68
    nonallergic adverse reactions to,
        62–64, 66
formaldehyde, 106, 117, 121, 122,
    141–42
fragrances, 116, 120–21
Frogskin, 116
Fulvicin, 151
fungi, 17, 31
Furadantin, 81, 83

gamma globulins, 6, 80, 168
Gantanol, 82
Gantrisin, 82, 84, 151
gastroesophageal reflux, 51
geraniol, 121
Germall 115, 117
gloves
    latex, 103–6, 168
    protective, 98, 101, 158
glutaraldehyde, 122
gnats, 131–32
goblet cells, 46
griseofulvin, 151
Gris-Peg, 151

hair dyes and sprays, 106, 109, 122
hair-waving preparations, 41
halogenated salicylanalides, 107,
    150
halothane, 84
Hashimoto's thyroiditis, 161
hay fever, 4, 5, 7–8, 73, 199
    food allergies and, 65, 69

as misleading term, 13
    See also seasonal allergic rhinitis
heliotrope rash, 159
henna, 109
HEPA, 33, 34, 42
hiatal hernias, 51
Hismanal, 22, 77, 78, 194
histamine, 5–6, 14–15, 108, 140, 167
histamine poisoning, 64
hives. See urticaria
Hollister Moisture Barrier, 101
horse allergies, 39
house mites. See mites
humidifiers, 33
hyaluronidase, 129
hydralazine, 81
hydrocarbons, 141
hydrochlorothiazide, 83
HydroDIURIL, 83, 151
Hydropel, 101
hydroxychloroquine, 154
hydroxycitronellal, 121
hydroxyzine, 193
Hymenoptera, 128–31
hypersensitivity, 2–3, 6–7, 166
hypersensitivity pneumonitis, 145–47
hypertonic solutions, 95
hypoallergenic products, 93, 99, 112,
    118, 189
Hytone, 102, 124, 196

ibuprofen, 130
IDDM, 161–63
idiosyncratic reactions, 78
IgA antibodies, 6
IgE antibodies, 5–8, 24, 52, 66, 80, 87,
    90, 108, 110, 111, 148, 166–67, 169,
    184, 199
    RAST method of testing for, 41, 53,
        70, 90, 130, 169, 185–86
IgG antibodies, 6, 8, 24, 199
IgM antibodies, 8
Ilosone, 84
imidazolidine amphoteric surfactants,
    117
immediate reactions (Type I reactions),
    6–7

imidazolidinyl urea, 117, 121
immune-complex disease. *See* Type III
   reactions
immune system, 3–7, 9
   drug side effects and, 77
   types of drug-induced reactions in,
      80–81
immunoglobulins, 6
immunotherapy. *See* allergy shots
Imuran, 149, 160, 162
Indocin, 55, 84, 86, 154, 156
indomethacin, 84, 154
INH, 78, 81, 84
insects, 127–32
   bites of, 4, 131–32, 134–36
   fragments and excrement of, 27, 66,
      136
   stings from, 73, 128–31, 168, 171
insulin, 80, 90, 168
insulin-dependent (Type I) diabetes
      mellitus, 161–63
Intal, 58, 83, 192–94
intolerance, 10
intolerant skin syndrome, 115–18
intradermal tests, 53, 69, 88, 89, 130,
      169, 184–85
intradermal titration approach, 175
in vitro testing, 185
irritant contact dermatitis, 94–99,
      119–20
isocyanates, 146
isoeugenol, 121
isoniazid, 78, 81, 84

Jackson, Michael, 165
juvenile-onset diabetes, 162

kapok, 30
Kathon CG, 122
Keflex, 81, 82, 87
Kenalog, 164
ketoconazole, 78, 84, 179, 194
kidney reactions to drugs, 77, 84

Lac-Hydrin lotion, 99, 112, 113, 158
lactic acid, 66, 117
lactobacili, 77

lactose intolerance, 63
Lamisil, 178
lanolin, 122
Lasix, 77
late-phase reaction, 8
latex rubber dermatitis, 103–6
lidocaine, 89
lindane, 109, 134
linseed, 40–41
liver reactions to drugs, 77, 84, 86
Locoid, 102, 124, 196
loratidine, 22, 194
lupus, 153–54
lymph nodes, swollen, 84–85
lymphocytes, 4, 7, 9, 83
Lysol, 32

Malathion, 136
manometric tests, 158
Marax, 58
marijuana smoke, 54
mascara, 117
masks, 25, 43, 146
mast cells, 5, 7–8, 80, 166
Maxiflor, 196
MCI/MI, 122
MCS, 140–43
meat tenderizer, 130, 168
mediators, 4, 5, 8, 80
Medic Alert bracelet, 92, 169
Medrol, 59, 109, 197
melanocytes, 164
Mellaril, 84
menthol, 109
mepivicaine, 89
metabisulfites, 49, 54, 68
Metaprel, 57
metered dose inhalers, 57
methacrylate, 117, 122
methadone, 83
methdilazine, 193
methicillin, 84, 87
methotrexate, 83
methyldopa, 84
methylprednisolone, 197
MGP, 122
miconized titanium dioxide, 107

phenylephrine, 195
phenyl-propanolamine, 22
phenytoin, 78, 81, 83–85
phospholipase A, 129
photoallergic contact dermatitis (photo-
    contact dermatitis), 82, 107–8, 147,
    149–50
photoallergies, 147–51
photopatch tests, 90, 107, 150, 190
photosensitivity reactions, 147
phototesting, 148, 149
phototoxic reactions, 82, 147
pineapple, 63
piperadines, 193
piprazines, 193
piroxicam, 151
plasma cells, 4, 5, 7
platelets, drug reactions of, 81, 85
PMLE, 147, 148–49
pneumonitis, hypersensitivity, 145–47
poison ivy, 4, 7, 9, 100–2, 164
pollens, 4, 17–20, 49, 184
    ragweed, 7–8, 17, 199
polymorphous light eruption (PMLE),
    147, 148–49
polymyositis, 159–60
Polysorbate 20, 117
polyurethane foam, 146
potassium hydroxide, 119
potassium sulfite, 68
PPD screening test, 53
PPL, 88
prazosin, 158
prednisolone, 59
prednisone, 24, 59, 72–73, 102, 109, 136,
    146, 149, 154, 156, 171, 197
Pre-pen, 88
prick test, 88, 89, 109
Primatine "P," 58
procainamide, 81, 83
procaine, 89
progressive systemic sclerosis (PSS),
    156–59
Pronestyl, 81, 83
propionic acid, 146
propylene glycol, 81, 117
propylthioiuracil, 81, 84

Proventil, 57
prunes, 63
pseudoephedrine, 22, 195
pseudomembranous colitis, 78
psoralens, 165
PSS, 156–59
pulmonary edema, 83
pulmonary function studies, 53–54
puncture tests, 53
purpura, 77
PUVA, 165
pyrethrin, 35, 134–36
Pyribenzamene, 193
pyrogens, 83

quackery, 172–81
quarternium 15, 106, 121
quaternary ammonium compounds,
    117
Quinaglute, 81, 83, 151
quinidine, 81, 83, 151
quinine, 81

radio-contrast media, allergies to, 91
radioimmunoassay, 185
radionics, 176
Randolph, Theron, 176–77
RAST, 41, 53, 70, 90, 130, 169, 185–86
Raynaud's phenomenon, 157, 158
respiratory tract
    drug reactions in, 83
    hypersensitivity pneumonitis, 145–47
    infections of, in asthma, 52
Revson, Charles, 180
rheumatic fever, acute, 152
rheumatoid arthritis, 155–56
rheumatoid factor test, 155–56
rhinitis
    food allergies and, 65
    medicamentosa, 23, 195
    seasonal allergic, 13–25
    vasomotor, 15–16
rhinitis-sinusitis-polyposis-asthma syn-
    drome, 86
rhinoconjunctivitis, allergic, 13
Rhizopus, 27
RID spray, 35, 135